Mama Is Still Here!

A mother and son's love passage through Alzheimer's

disease with daily prayers and devotionals

by

Norris Lee Roberts Jr. Ed.D.

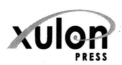

xulon
PRESS

Mama Is Still Here!
by Norris Lee Roberts Jr. Ed.D.

Printed in the United States of America

ISBN 9781625094728

Cover Illustration by Yana Simeonova

Contributing Editors: Christal Foster, Dr. Candance L. Virgil, Dr. JoAnn B. Clay, and Dr. Jeannie E. Roberts

Author's photograph by Ronald E. Haynes of Haynes Studios

www.xulonpress.com
www.norrislrobertsjr.com

*P*rofessional assistance for caregivers and families experiencing the daily ups and downs of Alzheimer's disease is being provided – free of charge – to the readers of Mama Is Still Here. If you're looking for Alzheimer's care or resources in your area, please call (888) 723-8241 to speak with a professional senior living advisor.

SeniorAdvisor.com, the nation's largest reviews and ratings source, helps millions of consumers every year find the best resources and senior care for their loved ones. Understanding how overwhelming the process can be – especially for loved ones with Alzheimer's disease or dementia – SeniorAdvisor.com is donating $250 to the Alzheimer's Association each time a family moves into a senior community in the trusted SeniorAdvisor.com network.*

This program is designed to be a simple way to raise money for Alzheimer's research, while simultaneously providing an accessible outlet for those most impacted by Alzheimer's disease to help fight it – by sharing this resource with their friends and family.

If you or someone you love could benefit from this service, please call (888) 723-8241. Together, we can help eradicate Alzheimer's disease.

Dedications

I provide a special dedication of this book to my mama, Daisy Dorothy Roberts, who is now in the grips of Alzheimer's disease, yet is handling it with grace and faith. Thank you, Mama, for planting the thought of sharing your story by simply saying with conviction on Thanksgiving Day, 2011, "Mama is still here!" Those words resonated in my spirit and my mind like an echo in a wide-open space surrounded by hills.

My mother's journey has been an incredible story, and I feel obligated to share it with the world. Mama has been a wonderful mother, wife, and dear friend. Thank you, Mama, for your continuous love, generosity, wisdom, and encouragement. I am eternally grateful to God for you. I also dedicate this book to my daddy, Norris Lee Roberts Sr., who encouraged me to continue writing. I thank him for giving me his blessings for writing not only Mama's story, but also their collective story.

I thank my wife, Dr. Jeannie Ellen Roberts, for being my supportive helpmate through the duration of this project, and for traversing this journey with me as I have experienced various emotions as I learned to cope. I also thank everyone who encouraged me, lifted me, counseled me, and otherwise contributed to the development of this work. Lastly, I dedicate this book to those who suffer, directly or indirectly, the effects of Alzheimer's disease. Caregivers, family members, friends, and others are in my thoughts and prayers, as are those who must endure the physical and mental effects of being victim to this insidious disease. I wrote this book to encourage you all;

we must help one another if by no other means than to say we understand, and to truly have compassion when someone says, "Today is a good day." Continue to pray for me as I continue the Alzheimer's journey with my mama.

Table of Contents

Introduction xv

Chapter 1: My Name Is Daisy! 23
Chapter 2: Sometimes You Have to Cry 29
Chapter 3: Turning Point 36
Chapter 4: It's a Family Affair 41
Chapter 5: Death at a Funeral 48
Chapter 6: Stranger in My House 51
Chapter 7: Before I Let Go 54
Chapter 8: 911 Emergency 57
Chapter 9: You Belong to Me 61
Chapter 10: Anniversary 64
Chapter 11: Lost without You 69
Chapter 12: Dancing Up a Storm! 72
Chapter 13: Mirror, Mirror, Mirror 76
Chapter 14: It Is Just My Imagination Running Away with Me 80
Chapter 15: Safe House 85
Chapter 16: The Water 89
Chapter 17: Coconut Cake 92
Chapter 18: The Invisible Children 97
Chapter 19: Weary and Burdened 100
Chapter 20: Happy Birthday 104
Chapter 21: Zoom 110

In Closing 113
Bible Versus 119

Foreword: Changed But Not Gone

"I cannot perform my role as wife, mother, sister, aunt or friend in the ways I did before. Yet I am still here. I am still all those things."
    —*Daisy*

*L*ike so many other tragic circumstances in life, seeing a loved one suffer from Alzheimer's feels deeply personal, but involves struggles that are universal. In *Mama Is Still Here!*, Norris Lee Roberts Jr. writes about his mother's experience with the disease now plaguing five million people in the United States captures both sides of the struggle.

Throughout the book, we gain a clear picture of who Daisy (the Mama in question) is. A great cook with a special skill for making coconut cake, the "family's memory maker," a doting mother and a loving wife; the woman at the center of the story shines through even as she sometimes fails to recognize those parts of herself.

With this book, Roberts both celebrates all the things that make his mother special, while at the same painting a clear picture of the challenges most Alzheimer's patients and their families face. For anyone who doesn't know what to expect from an Alzheimer's diagnosis, the book covers many of the basics:

- The early days of denial, misdiagnosis and trying to cover the symptoms of the disease up.
- The shock, disbelief, and "why me" sense of despair when the Alzheimer's diagnosis finally comes.

- All the little things that the Alzheimer's patient can no longer do and needs help with – from cooking and running errands in the early days to getting dressed and bathing herself in the later days.
- The techniques caregivers must figure out to work around the problems Alzheimer's causes. Roberts recounts scenes of distracting his mother from her despair by telling old family stories, and easing transitions from one place to another by making them as quick as possible.
- The abandonment of many friends and family members who find visiting too uncomfortable. "Fear drove people away," explains Daisy.
- The violence and anger some patients exhibit, in spite of always having been gentle and non-violent in their lives before Alzheimer's.
- The rare moments of lucidity that allow an Alzheimer's patient who has seemed long gone for months to suddenly be fully present for a family celebration or significant moment with a loved one.
- The constant struggles and re-arrangements of every day life that caregivers must make to accommodate the illness and help their loved one get through it with as little suffering as possible.

Roberts recounts all these experiences as they played out in his family and describes the emotional toll they often took. But he also takes care to emphasize the moments when his mother was more present as her usual self, and how much more valuable to him, his father, and the rest of the family those times were because of the challenges they'd faced. He starts off each chapter with an inspiring quote, and ends it with a relevant scripture and prayer in the hopes of giving the reader something they can use to get through the hardest times.

The familiar experiences for Alzheimer's patients and the emotions they provoke in the people they love come through clearly. For anyone reeling from a recent diagnosis of their own, wondering what to expect in the days to come for a loved one in the early stages, or just looking to hear that someone else has dealt with what they're going through – this book can provide catharsis, guidance, and the feeling that you're not alone.

—Review by Kristen Hicks, writer for SeniorAdvisor.com, the nation's largest ratings and reviews site for Alzheimer's care

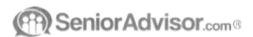

SeniorAdvisor.com is the premier consumer ratings and reviews site for senior care providers across the US and Canada. The innovative website provides easy access to the information families need when making a senior living decision, and features trusted reviews and advice from local residents and their loved ones. SeniorAdvisor.com brings functionality and convenience to a process that tends to be complex and overwhelming. SeniorAdvisor/com is an independent operating unit of **A Place for Mom, Inc.**

Webite at www.SeniorAdvisor.com
Blog at http://blog.senioradvisor.com
Twitter at http://twitter.com/SeniorAdvisor
Google+ at google.com/+Senioradvisor

Introduction

Find a place inside where there's joy,
and the joy will burn out the pain.
—Joseph Campbell

This book is for Alzheimer's sufferers, caregivers, and their loved ones. Alzheimer's is a fatal inflammatory degenerative brain disease that causes a gradual decline in brain activity. Over an approximate period of ten years, sufferers progressively lose various forms of memory, culminating in a vegetative state before death. At each leg of this arduous journey, loved ones fall victim to sufferers' loss of special memories, recognition, and simple blessings, such as smiles, acknowledgement, or a warm touch. In the early stages of Alzheimer's, symptoms are inconsistent and unpredictable, which makes diagnosis difficult. Once symptoms become more consistent and predictable, and the disease has progressed to moderate stages, brain function decline is noticeable and undeniable.

My mama, Daisy Dorothy Roberts, has Alzheimer's disease. Mama's was diagnosed once the disease had progressed to the moderate stage. Initially, learning Mama had Alzheimer's was unbelievable and inconceivable to me. I wanted to know the probable causes and available treatments. I wanted to learn as much as I could, so I could better support our family's trial or fight with Alzheimer's. I was more than willing to go into battle for her.

As I learned more about the disease and the unfortunate prognosis, I felt overwhelmed by fear and utter disappointment. The diagnosis seemed unfair to me because Mama had always taken good care of herself. She carefully monitored her diet and always incorporated exercise and activity into her daily routine. Mama lived by and believed in Benjamin Franklin's famous quote, "An ounce of prevention is worth a pound of cure," and instilled it in her family.

After the diagnosis, sometimes I would torture myself with the ultimate question, "How could this have happened to her?" Finally, I cried out to God in prayer. I asked God to remove the spirit of fear from my heart, to help me move forward, and to help me ride the waves of my overwhelming emotions. Through prayer and thanksgiving, I asked God for His peace and His wisdom for all things yet to come with Mama's Alzheimer's disease. As the head of my household, I also knew I had to be strong not only for my mama, but for my own family. I wondered if I would be able to manage it all and divest my feelings from what to do for Mama's sake. *The journey begins now*, I thought.

Included in this book are collections of twenty-one stories reflecting upon Mama's life before and after her Alzheimer's diagnosis, along with devotionals and prayers. Each story begins with a secular quote, and each story ends with a scripture quote from the Bible and a prayer from my heart. The scriptures and prayers are words of encouragement, and words of challenging and inspiring thoughts centered on the Christian faith. It is my hope that the collections of scriptures and prayers I was inspired to include will help those confronted with the disease to move to a more peaceful acceptance, and develop a greater understanding of the unparalleled world of Alzheimer's.

According to the Alzheimer's Association, an estimated five million Americans have Alzheimer's, and the number is growing. I am a Christian, and believe the Word of God can provide healing and peace for Alzheimer's sufferers, their caregivers, and their loved ones. The progression of Alzheimer's is relentlessly persistent; it challenges one's endurance, strength, and faith with little or no pause. My daily prayer is to ask God to help me trust him for everything and doubt him for nothing.

I have observed Mama's progression from the moderate stages of the Alzheimer's to the more severe stages. Initially, I struggled with grief and the spirit of fear. According to Elisabeth Kubler-Ross

(2005), there are five stages of grief: denial, anger, bargaining, depression, and acceptance. Spouses, children, grandchildren, siblings, other family members, and friends experience the five stages of loss and grief. According to Dr. Elaine R Axelrod (2012), we all move back and forth through the various stages of loss and grief before coming to acceptance with peace. The grieving process is not sequential; it is a reiterative process.

I was not prepared to deal with the loss and grief because I did not understand or believe that this could be happening to someone as wonderful and dear as my mother. The fear and anxiety of the constant unknown exasperated me. I felt like I would go berserk when I received a call from my parents. The overwhelming spirit of fear and panic distracted me and I could not focus on a solution. Series of preemptive tragedies flooded my mind. I prayed to the Lord for peace, courage, and strength to make sense of my mother's disease and its affect on me and my family. I asked him to give me a sense of calm so I could carry on. God answered my prayers, but I must continue to vigilantly renew my mind and fortify my faith: "Let this mind be in you, which was also in Christ Jesus" (Phil. 2:5 KJV). I prayed to the Lord to remove the spirit of fear from my mind when Daddy or Mama's sister, Aunt Mary Ann, telephoned me. I trusted God would give me the strength and courage to conquer my fears and anxiety—and he has.

There is a terrible stigma and prejudice against people with Alzheimer's and their families. Family, friends, and acquaintances visit and interact with the caregiver and the Alzheimer's sufferer less and less over time. People stay away because the effects of the disease make them feel uncomfortable, or they do not want to see the Alzheimer's sufferer out of sorts. This detachment from people is the beginning of social isolation, which is a significant barrier to the well-being of individuals with Alzheimer's.

I hope these twenty-one stories and devotions can provide a greater awareness and more understanding and acceptance for Alzheimer's sufferers and their caregivers. The story "Turning Point" describes and reflects upon the variety of symptoms leading up to the Alzheimer's diagnosis. The first story, "My Name is Daisy!" is in Mama's voice, and the last story, "Zoom," is in her voice as well.

The other nineteen stories describe Mama's journey with Alzheimer's in my voice, providing the reader insight into Mama's upbringing, interests, and accomplishments before her Alzheimer's diagnosis.

I wrote this book for those who are also traveling on their own personal journeys with Alzheimer's disease, but writing this book also helped me cope with the ever-changing dynamic that has become part of my daily life. I have tried to adapt to what is currently taking place, but I also have had to allow for, and adjust to, those changes that are yet to come. I juggle numerous responsibilities and continue to realize personal goals. However, each day I have this enormous elephant in the room called Alzheimer's disease that demands its own portion of my attention, energy, authority, and control. Writing this book was, therefore, cathartic for me; it rejuvenated my faith and confirmed my belief that God truly takes care of one's pain, suffering, and fear and helps one find peace in situations where peace could not normally exist. As I continue in my journey, I am encouraged by the vision of putting one foot in front of the other, as Mama would want me to do.

I feel I must clarify why I refer to my mother as "Mama" and my father as "Daddy" throughout this book. First of all, I am comfortable calling them these terms. In addition, they have both earned these titles. There is a definite difference between what may seem to be interchangeable terms for parents. Mothers and fathers are capable of bringing life into the world. When you have a Mama and a Daddy, however, you have two people who unconditionally, faithfully, and eternally love you, support you, encourage you, and teach you to the best of their abilities. You share a relationship with your parents like no other in the universe. They "get" you on every level, and many times, they know your dreams, fears, and trials better than you do. They understand a simple look or a modest gesture, and return it with a communication only a privileged few could ever share. The relationship is serious to me, and it is absolute. I also love these people unconditionally, faithfully, and eternally. I am also doing my best to support and encourage them, and to show them that I appreciate all they have done for me. I am so thankful to God to have a Mama and a Daddy, and not just a mother and father.

At the time of this writing, Mama and Daddy have been married for forty-eight years. God bless them both. God bless Daddy, for he has honored Mama by being a husband and the head of the household. Daddy has exhibited and modeled what it means to honor the marriage vow, "for better or for worse." It is difficult for me to imagine how Alzheimer's could get any worse.

I have one sister, Iris, who is four years younger than I am and is married with three boys: Rodney II, Bradley, and Emory. I have been married to Jeannie Ellen for twenty-three years. We have two twin children, Norris Lee III and Jeannie Nicole, and we are grandparents to two beautiful baby girls named Khloe Nicole and Zoe Diane.

Mama and Daddy's first home was a four-family flat on Northland Avenue in North St. Louis. The owners were Daddy's Great Aunt Dee Shelton and Great Uncle Ruben Shelton from Daddy's side of the family. Aunt Dee and Uncle Ruben lived two doors down, and we saw them frequently. They migrated from Mississippi in the years before to seek a better standard of living and greater opportunity. What I remembered most about this house was the big tree with red apples in the backyard and the clotheslines. Mama used to hang our wash on the line to dry. The yard was fenced in and backed to an alley behind, where garbage trucks picked up trash each week. Aunt Dee had a vegetable garden in the back of the flat. She had roses, violets, and mums planted throughout the perimeter of the yard. This is where I played and rode my bike in the early years of my life.

Mama and Daddy were very much a team when it came to providing for our little family. Mama and Daddy both worked; I was always with one of them. Daddy worked second shift at General Motors and Mama worked for Saint Louis Public Schools as a teacher. Working different shifts enabled Mama and Daddy to care for us without using day care services, and they were able to share one car. Daddy would take Mama to work, and he would keep the car all day and later pick Mama up from work. Mama would then drop Daddy off at work, and she would keep the car. Daddy would get a ride back from either his brother, brother-in-law, cousins, or friends. Daddy had a tremendous work ethic, and he was able to get many relatives jobs at General Motors. They all eventually retired from General Motors.

There was always lots of family around when I was growing up, and all of our family went to Hopewell Baptist Church every Sunday. My great-grandparents, Mama Cornelia and Papa Thomas, Daddy's grandparents on his mother's side, were the first of our family to attend. After church, we would have dinner at home and later visit relatives' homes. Mama and Daddy always stayed connected with family.

My sister, Iris Antonia, was born when I was four years old. She was Mama's hope, dream, and prayer; Mama wanted a little girl because she already had a little boy. Mama was a Southern mother; mothers in the South seem to agonize over what to name their baby more than giving birth. Mama wanted her daughter to have a flower name, and she came up with Iris. The name Iris was a strong name with a history dating back to Ancient Greek times and the deep purple Iris denoted royalty and was one of Mama's most favorite colors. Antonia is the name of a town in Jefferson County, Missouri. We traveled to Mississippi often, and Mama would always call out the name of the town as we drove by. She expressed how she liked the name and believed it would be a wonderful middle name for a girl. Mama loved having a little girl to dress up; Mama would often make Iris and herself matching dresses, and they would wear them to church and family gatherings.

Mama and Daddy's many sacrifices in the first ten years of their marriage paid off well. Because they had saved, they were able to buy another car. They began to acquire some of the luxuries of life. Daddy showered Mama with gifts, such as furs, coats, and jewelry. In the seventies, we had a TV in every room of our apartment, and we owned multiple phones. Mama and Daddy raised my sister and me to be accustomed to having nice things. Mama and Daddy were the trendsetters in the family. They often introduced their siblings to new ideas and innovations.

Daddy worked full-time at General Motors and part-time as a mechanic at Western Auto. Mama taught full-time at Saint Louis Public Schools. My sister and I both attended a parochial school, Holy Rosary, on Margareta Avenue. After ten years of living in a four-family flat on Northland Avenue, Mama and Daddy purchased their first and only home, a three-bedroom with two bathrooms in

North Saint Louis County. Our family had shifted from urban living to suburban living. Mama loved suburban living; my sister and I were involved in multiple activities, including ones at our church. Iris began synchronized skating, track and field, girl scouts, piano, flute, and debutantes balls. I became involved in track and field, skating, boy scouts, piano, and trombone. Mama and Daddy provided us with an outstanding upbringing.

My sister and I both graduated from high school and college, and we both married shortly after college. Iris and I both fulfilled our parents' hopes and dreams for us, and this made Mama very proud. I was the first to get married and the first to have children; the first grandchildren were fraternal boy and girl twins. This was an exciting time for Mama and Daddy; becoming grandparents to twins was very special to them both, but especially to Daddy because he was a twin. Daddy's twin sister's name is Nancy Ann. Mama and Daddy enjoyed spoiling their grandchildren and even took them on trips out of state, including to Mississippi. Mama and Daddy had significant time and discretionary income and enjoyed spending time and money on their grandchildren. At this time they were forty-eight years young.

Chapter 1:

My Name Is Daisy!

When you deal with a person who is experiencing dementia,
you can see where they're struggling with knowledge.
You can see what they forget completely, what they forget
but they know what they once knew.
You can tell how they're trying to remember.
—Walter Mosley

The following excerpt is from the author's mother: My name is Daisy, and I am in between the later to severe stages of Alzheimer's disease. At first, I never considered or believed that I had acquired Alzheimer's. I am not sure when my symptoms began; however, I did recognize that something was not quite right. I know most people misplace things such as keys or a purse every now and then. We all get confused or lost in areas we do not frequently travel. Initially, my memory was only impaired occasionally; the memory loss or confusion would happen from time to time in spells. When I could not account for what had happened prior to my memory lapse, I was frustrated. I did not interpret any of my symptoms to be anything serious. I figured it was just the effects of menopause and getting older. Unfortunately, I was wrong!

Initially, I was misdiagnosed with clinical depression, and my doctor prescribed Lexapro, which made me feel lethargic and sleepy, not to mention the diarrhea. I stopped taking the medication; I just figured I would cope with my depression on my own. This diagnosis concerned me, but it did not devastate me. I felt depression was a treatable diagnosis and it would soon pass. Yet the diagnosis did not explain my intermittent memory lapses.

In the meantime, I used my grandchildren to help me get around town. This was easy; I would ask my son or my daughter-in-law to drop the grandchildren off, and I used them as my human navigation systems. This really worked out great for a while; I kept my independence, and I was able to spend time with my grandchildren. I blamed my directional challenges on the significant highway construction throughout the St. Louis metropolitan area.

After learning of my true diagnosis, I often cried out to God with tears in my eyes. I asked the Lord, "Why me? Why can't the doctors cure me? I felt I was losing myself in every way. I sometimes asked God to give me another disease like cancer, something I could fight.

After wallowing in self-pity, I finally began to remember many of the things I was grateful for, and I appreciated my life a bit more. I remembered having a tumor the size of a grapefruit surgically removed while my children were in college. Then I reflected on the Bible story of Lazarus's resurrection, and I thought about how there was no second resurrection. If my tumor had been malignant, I would have had to undergo chemotherapy and radiation. "What if?" Then I begin to thank the Lord for how he blessed me with such a wonderful life.

I came to realize that suffering was a part of life. There would be trials, and I was in my greatest trial of my life. I thanked the Lord for allowing me to be a part of my grandchildren's lives after surgeons removed the tumor. I enjoyed being a grandmother. My grandchildren and I truly had a blast! We had many adventures traveling, shopping, and eating out. They were spoiled, and I enjoyed spoiling them.

Because my Alzheimer's was not diagnosed until I was in the mid-stage, I spent much of the time in the early onset of the disease lost in frustration, anxiety, and confusion. I was not happy, and I blamed every problem on my husband, Norris. I wanted him to carry my pain of feeling helpless due to my memory lapses. We both were frustrated with the problem, and neither of us wanted to believe this was happening to me. My experience reminded me of the Gladys Knight song "Neither One of Us." Having Alzheimer's is like a long good-bye. Norris and I had our differences of opinions, and Alzheimer's amplified our differences. I know it was exhausting for him, but he weathered through it with me.

Sometimes I caught myself not making any sense in my conversations. I knew I was repeating myself a lot. My sister, Mary Ann, and my daughter, Iris, would often call me on things I may have said five minutes ago. I would cover it by joking or distracting them with questions. I don't believe I was intentionally trying to throw them off; I think my denial of any problem was my way to maintain control and independence.

There was no consistency or predictability to the memory lapses and the impaired memory loss and confusion. I became confused in familiar places I frequented quite often. One of my favorite pastimes, shopping, became difficult. Since I was afraid I would have a memory lapse while I was out shopping, I began to use the "Home Shopping Network" instead. I would also get lost driving to the grocery store, and once I was even lost in the grocery store. At times, I thought I was going crazy. So I sent others to get items I needed from the store.

I over-paid some bills and did not pay other bills at all. Many of my daily activities started to become a struggle, including sewing, cooking, and putting on my makeup. I never would have thought feeling pretty would be a struggle for me. I started to forget how to do things I had done easily for more than forty years. These frustrations led to mood and personality changes.

I would often call my children by any name but their own. I called my daughter, Iris, by my sister's name. I would call my son, Junior, by many names, such as one of my many younger brothers' names. First I would call him Howard, then I would call him Bo, and then he was George or Thomas. I did this so much that they started to answer to any name I called them. I would joke with my sister and say,

"They know who I am talking to."

Throughout this mid-stage, I would say many of the following phrases often out of context:

"Hmm! How did I get here? I don't remember coming to this place."

"Norris, where are you?"

"I'm freezing! Aren't you cold?"

"Norris, why don't you answer me? You are not supposed to leave me!"

"I misplaced those damn car keys again!"

"I've got to get out of here; I want to go home to my Mama and Daddy!"

"I have to see about the children; they are hungry!"

"The next time he touches me, I am going to kill him!"

"Don't touch me, and I mean it!"

"What the hell is going on here?"

"This house is a mess...Oh, there you are!"

"Norris, answer me."

"Where is that girl?"

"I want to see my mother and father!"

"Who is that? You scared me! What did you say?"

"Hmm! Who is this person combing my hair?"

"No one cares about me; I am going to kill myself!"

"I recognized him, but I can't seem to recall his name."

"Huh?"

Now I am at a more severe stage of Alzheimer's, and I require assistance with all activities of daily living. My husband, Norris, is my full-time, primary caregiver. Sometimes I find it remarkable that he has stood by me for this long. He has truly surprised me as a husband. I did not know he had it in him. Lord knows he had to reach deep to acquire the level of patience and kindness needed to take care of me in this condition. Yet, he did it!

Now I cannot always control my bowels and bladder. I never would have expected my memory to decline to the point that I would not know to sit on the toilet. I am a private and modest woman. I hate not being able to shower or bathe myself, and I have not gotten used to others doing these kinds of things for me.

I know there is a lot I have forgotten; I just do not know what it all is anymore. The best way to describe my memory is like Swiss cheese! The memory lapses, or the Swiss cheese holes, have increased significantly as the disease has progressed. I often find myself lost in my memories. The past and the present are a continuous blur. In spite of it all, my memory problems have not stopped me from wanting, which is the only form of independence I have left. When I am not in a memory lapse, I do recognize how my family and friends have truly struggled with my illness.

As my Alzheimer's disease progressed, relatives and friends avoided or feared me. This behavior shocked my husband and children, but not me. I knew it would happen, and that is why I did not share my diagnosis freely with family and friends in the early on-set. Fear drove people away.

I do sense the heartache and the pain around me. I believe what bothers family and friends the most is my inability to recognize them or myself and my inability to communicate with them in a two-sided conversation. They do not realize that I do understand more than they think. "I am still here!" I cry out. I try to give them signs to let them know I do understand. "I am still here!" Most of all, I want them to know that I love them.

There are some people I am able to connect with spiritually. I have the strongest spiritual connection with my son. He is able to bring me back to the present when I have slipped deep into my long-term memories. He sometimes brings me back just by moving me to my seat at the kitchen table. I think he calls my seat position at the kitchen table seven o'clock. Combing my hair is another thing that brings me back to the present. I am very happy my son can stand in the gap for me when I am lost between the past and the present.

With Alzheimer's we all have to dig deep. I cannot perform my role as wife, mother, sister, aunt, or friend in the ways I did before. Yet, I am still here. I am still all those things, and I perform them all to the best of my ability. In spite of all we have endured as a family, I have not given up. "Mama is still here!"

Scripture Help: "I tell you the truth, when you were younger you dressed yourself and went where you wanted; but when you are old you will stretch out your hands, and someone else will dress you and lead you where you do not want to go. Jesus said this to indicate the kind of death by which Peter would glorify God. Then he said to him, 'Follow me!'"(John 21:18–19 NIV).

Prayer: Heavenly Father, thank you! Hear my prayer for my suffering. My days are now filled with fear and confusion. And in the days when memory has gone, Lord, I ask you to give me peace in my heart to endure this trial. Lord, thank you for giving me the dignity I desperately want and desire in this time of life. Lord, I ask you to shower all members of my family with blessings, hope, and greater love. Thank you, Lord, for all the ways you have blessed my family and me. Thank you for being our all when we have no clue what to do next. We are lost in many ways, yet we look to you as our guide, our teacher, and our comforter! Thank you, Lord. In Jesus' name, I pray. Amen.

Chapter 2:

Sometimes You Have to Cry

If you haven't cried, your eyes can't be beautiful.
—Sophia Loren

It was a cloudy and gloomy day in Saint Louis. I was out and about, running errands, when my cell phone rang. It was Daddy. He called my name, and immediately I knew he was stressed. I asked, "Are you okay?" He hesitated with a sigh of relief. Then he replied, "I am OK, but Daisy is crying. She is crying a lot! I cannot get her to stop. I do not know what to do." I replied, "I am on my way!"

I drove to their house. When I rang the doorbell, there was no answer, so I let myself in. I called for Mama and Daddy hesitantly. Daddy walked into the living room and answered my call. "I am glad you are here. Daisy has been crying, and I can't get her to stop. I do not know if she is in pain or what. She wants to go home to her mother and father. I tried to tell Daisy that her mother, Mama Mary, died some time ago. And you know her father, Papa Johnnie, is in a nursing home."

I could tell Daddy was at his wit's end. I suggested he leave the house to take a break. With a smile on his face and a look of relief, Daddy grabbed his hat and jacket and left in his truck as though he were escaping from a burning building. I smiled as I looked out the dining room window and I watched him as he drove off. I was happy to give him a break. I went into the family room where Mama was sitting and wiping the tears from her eyes. When she saw me, she immediately called me Howard, which is her younger brother's name. I did not correct Mama; I had learned from previous experiences that correcting her made her more upset. I went along with the person she believed I was in the moment. Mama pleaded with me to drive her home; she wanted to be with her mother and father. After she pleaded and bargained with me for more than ten minutes, she began to cry uncontrollably.

It was sad and painful to see Mama cry. I could not give her what she wanted, and I felt her agony. I decided that I needed to distract her from where she was mentally. I led Mama to the kitchen table, to the place where she had sat since I was a little boy, at seat position seven o'clock. She had shared so much with me in this spot. Being seated there seemed to calm Mama down and return her to the present.

Sitting at the kitchen table with her brought back many memories for me. I began to reflect on all I knew about Mama's childhood. I reflected on Mama's life in Mississippi, and I began to share her story with her. I became the storyteller, and Mama patiently listened.

Mama, Daisy Dorothy Phillips Roberts, was born August 29, 1940 in Winona, Mississippi, the sixth child of Johnnie Phillips and Mary Henson Phillips. In their large family of three daughters and eight sons, Daisy was a warm, giving, and energetic girl, who was devoted to her siblings and parents. The family first lived in rural Kilmichael, Mississippi. They later moved to the Campbell Hill area in Winona Mississippi. The family finally settled at a small farm on the outer perimeter of Winona off New Hope Road. For many years, family members would congregate at this family home to spend quality time.

Mama was a wonderful and joyful individual. She was filled with hope, generosity, and love. Mama always exuded positive energy, and many were attracted to her light. In the small community where she grew up, Mama was adored; she readily and happily helped neighbors and friends. Mama had an amazing spirit to serve others, and this brought her great joy and made her so special in the eyes of family and friends. Mama was a gracious and charming host; she had a way of making everyone feel welcome.

Mama shared many stories about her childhood in Mississippi from her favorite seat at the kitchen table. The first house Mama lived in did not have running water. Several years after she was born, the family upgraded to a house that only had running water at the kitchen sink. Mama would share stories about cooking on a wood stove. She also shared stories of how she had to share one bed with two sisters. Mama talked about the long list of chores each of her brothers did daily and how far away they lived from town. Since local town entertainment was not a consideration, she and her siblings entertained themselves with games, singing, and making their chores fun. As I thought about Mama's childhood, I recalled my own experiences of this family farm. As a young boy, I would watch my uncles and grandparents work with the animals. They killed chickens and slaughtered hogs and cows, and milked cows. Kids helped by picking fruit and, together with the fresh meat, hauled it to the house. My grandmother, mother, and aunts transformed these items into sumptuous meals. This collective approach to work seemed comfortable, logical, and allowed each person to take part in the family rewards at the table. I never could believe how much food was left over, even after all were satisfied. I believe those memories have given my life balance and understanding. I am very thankful to my mother for allowing me to share in those experiences, and for teaching me along the way that families work together.

As I reflected on her childhood stories, I was struck by the difference from what I always knew as a boy who shared a household with a single sibling and parents who worked outside the home. I enjoyed the same things most boys my age enjoyed, such as riding a bike and buying candy at the local store. I had a few brief chores to do, but mainly I was free to enjoy life every day and all it had to offer. Life in the forties and fifties in rural Mississippi was indeed very challenging and different from the life I led as a child in the sixties and seventies in the Midwest.

One of Mama's fondest memories she would always share around Christmastime was when she was a little girl and it snowed. Mama Millie, Mama's great-grandmother on her mother's side of the family, would tell the girls how to make ice cream with snow. They would go up on the roof to get the snow. Then they would mix the snow with milk, sugar, and vanilla in a bowl.

Mama would share four amazing facts about Mama Millie. First, Mama Millie was eight years old when the slaves were set free after the civil war. Second, Mama Millie lived to be one hundred and fourteen years old. Third, Mama Millie went blind in her eighties because she had untreated glaucoma. And fourth, Mama Millie outlived all of her children. Mama recalled that Mama Millie died when Mama was in high school, but many of the lessons she taught her continued to live on. Mama felt that by telling Mama Millie's story, a part of her would continue to live on through her children and grandchildren, too.

Mama Mae Judy was Mama's grandmother on her mother's side of the family. Mama Mae Judy was an expert at making lye-soap. Because it was a dangerous process, Mama and her eldest sister, Aunt Mae Judy, would watch Mama Mae Judy make the soap from a window inside the house. Mama Mae Judy would build a big fire outside and use a huge pot the size of a barrel. Mama would watch her grandmother stir the bubbling pot with a broomstick while she wore safety goggles and rubber gloves.

Mama attended public schools and graduated in 1960 from Knox High School, a segregated high school in Winona. Mama often shared stories about how she played basketball, ran track, and sang in the high school choir. Dr. Winbush was the high school choir director and was Mama's most influential teacher. Mama described Dr. Winbush as an extraordinary man who was committed to encouraging excellence in each of his pupils. Mama often told stories about the variety of music the choir practiced and the many choir performances she participated in. Mama's favorite song was "Swing Low Sweet Chariot." When telling the story, Mama would occasionally sing a few bars of the song just to illustrate her point. I enjoyed hearing her sing and would often ask her to sing just a little bit more.

Mama also talked about her high school prom. She recalled how proud she was of the junior classmen who decorated the gym for the senior prom each year. And she described how much fun it was when she was finally able to participate. Mama also talked often about home economics, in which she formally learned how to sew. Sewing was one of Mama's passions, and she became an excellent tailor. Through the years, Mama was able to do everything from alterations to designing originals for herself and my sister, Iris.

For Mama's father, Papa Johnnie, employment came from a variety of jobs, such as driving a truck or a bus; however, the farm was always a vital part of the family's budget. Producing their own food saved them money, and the harvest provided another source of income. They raised chickens, cows, and pigs, and they grew a variety of fruits and vegetables, such as peas, greens, okra, green beans, sweet potatoes, corn, cucumbers, butter beans, sugar canes, apples, peanuts, plums, peaches, cantaloupes, and watermelons.

After her graduation from high school, Mama pursued an education in business at Mississippi Vocational College at Itta Bena, Mississippi. Mama graduated in 1964 and initially wanted to use her degree to obtain a position as an office manager or administrative assistant. After moving to St. Louis, she continued to see herself as a "career gal." She was disappointed to realize, though, that employers preferred to hire single women with no college education for secretarial positions. And, of course, employers would prefer whites to coloreds in the segregated South, even though they would not come right out and say this. Corporate employers would suggest Mama teach instead, since she had a degree. Mama always thought it was a nice way of saying they were not hiring colored women for those positions. After interviewing for a position as an executive secretary at a local manufacturing plant, Mama was offered a position to work as a third shift lineman, which was disappointing and insulting. Since family was Mama's focus, she realized the teaching profession afforded her to focus on her role as wife and mother.

Mama deeply loved her family, relatives, and close friends. Mama was determined to keep the family connected for the greater good, and she accomplished this through frequent trips to Mississippi and through her annual New Year's Day dinners. Mama always wanted everyone to begin the New Year together in celebration and thanksgiving with a feast. Mama also kept the family connected by inviting her nephews and nieces to spend parts of their summer with her in St. Louis.

Mama would also tell us funny or interesting stories about many events from her chair at the kitchen table positioned at 7 o'clock. I remember one tale about how Mama would sleepwalk when she was a child. Mama's mother, Mama Mary, would always wake her up before she walked out on the front porch. Because the sleepwalking was increasing and becoming more and more dangerous, Mama Mary consulted with the doctor about Mama's sleepwalking. The doctor instructed Mama Mary not to wake Mama up, but to let her sleepwalk to wherever she was going and then allow Mama to wake herself up. Mama Mary followed the doctor's advice. One night when Mama was sleepwalking again, Mama's eldest sister, Mae Judy, who shared a bed with her, got Mama Mary. Mama Mary and Uncle Edward followed Mama with a lantern to her destination. Uncle Edward wanted to wake her since they were getting a little far from the house. Mama Mary replied, "Let her be!" They quietly continue to follow her, being careful not to wake her. She walked more than 400 yards away from the house. She stopped at a tree on the edge of the hill with a steep drop-off into the dirt road below where she played everyday. Again, Uncle Edward wanted to wake her and again Mama Mary would not let him. Mama Mary said, "Hush!" They all stood still as Mama stayed there for more than a minute and then awakened. Finally, Mama woke up screaming, confused and frightened to find herself outside in the pitch dark. Uncle Edward grabbed her and carried back to the house. Since that awakening, Mama never walked in her sleep again.

Mama's older brothers were extraordinarily creative. They were only kids but were beyond their years in the areas of mechanics, electricity and wood working. At the time, Mama was the youngest and smallest and was often used as a guinea pig or test dummy for many of her brothers and older sister's projects, such as go-karts, miniature houses and furniture they would build. Her older brothers and sister made a slingshot out of a large tree and some stretchable, rubber like tubing to use as the firing mechanism. They released Mama from the slingshot, and she sailed through the air like a cannon ball. When she landed, Mama was knocked unconscious and suffered a severe head injury. Mama's father cut the slingshot down and whipped them for nearly killing their sister. He dared them to ever do anything like that again. Whenever Mama told the story, however, she would laugh as though she was recalling an episode from *The Three Stooges*. She loved to talk about how she and her siblings would get into the most unusual activities.

To me Mama is many things: a greatest teacher, role model, and listener. Maya Angelou once said, "I've learned people will forget what you said, people will forget what you did, but people will never forget how you made them feel" (BrainyQuote, 2012). I enjoyed reflecting on how Mama made me feel and how she made others feel throughout my life, and I love her even more for it. We sat together at the table and I held her hand. We both wandered down memory lane together. And in the following moments, she returned to me whole and at peace once again. Mama called me by name and asked for Daddy by name.

Scripture Help: "For I know the plans I have for you," declares the LORD, "plans to prosper you and not to harm you, plans to give you hope and a future" (Jer. 29:11 NIV).

Prayer: Lord, don't ignore the tears of Alzheimer's sufferers and their caregivers. Lord, please hear their cries for help and hear their silent thoughts. It is a difficult time they share and I thank you for the many times you have given us all help, always listening when we have called to you in our darkest moments. When all seemed to be lost, you are at our side. Lord, you always listen and you have always come to our rescue with comfort and guidance. Lord, change our mourning into dancing and singing. Lord, clothe us with your joy. I look forward to the day when every tear is wiped away. Until now, use our tears to make our weeping eyes beautiful, and full of hope and joy. In the holy name of Jesus, we pray. Amen.

Chapter 3:

Turning Point

Life is always at some turning point.
—Irwin Edman

After Daddy retired and was with Mama around the clock, Daddy could no longer deny Mama's memory problems. Mama's changes in mood and personality, confusion, and the inability to simply hand write a note with pen and paper were obvious. Something was wrong and he had to take the responsibility to find out. This cornered him to make an appointment for Mama to see her primary care physician, Dr. Jennings.

After the nurse escorted Mama, Daddy and my sister Iris to the examination room, they quietly waited in silence. Mama was seated on the examination table where the nurse took her vitals, Daddy was seated in the chair next to the examination table and Iris was seated in the chair on the same wall of the door. Dr. Jennings broke the silence with a polite knock and entered. "Hello, Ms. Daisy. How have you been? And hello Mr. Norris and I presumed this is your daughter." Iris replied, "Yes, I talked with you on the phone." Dr. Jennings, smiling pleasantly, replied, "Iris, pleased to meet you. Good morning to you all!" Mama and Daddy both politely replied, "Good Morning." Dr. Jennings was a tall white male, with broad shoulders and short brown hair with a little gray. Mama loved her soap operas. We sometimes joked the reason Mama liked Dr. Jennings so much was because he reminded her of one of the doctors she was fond of on the TV soap opera *General Hospital*. Dr. Jennings was familiar with Alzheimer's on a personal level. His father died of Alzheimer's a few years prior.

It was obvious that Dr. Jennings was fond of Mama and having to confirm what we all already knew was difficult for him. At the time of the examination, Mama was very confused. Dr. Jennings began the examination with a question. He said, "Daisy, what day of the week is it?" Mama chuckled and replied, "It is the day I came to the doctor's office." Dr. Jennings asked again, "Daisy, what day of the week is it? The right answer is Monday, Tuesday, Wednesday, Thursday, or Friday." Mama replied, "Huh, it is the day after yesterday." Dr. Jennings realized this was not going anywhere. Next Dr. Jennings asked slowly and calmly, "Daisy, who is President of the United States?" Mama replied, "Harry Truman." Dr. Jennings was surprised at her answer. He scratched his head and said, "Wow! That's an amazing answer." Under his breath, he said to Daddy, "I expected a more recent president, like Kennedy, Johnson, or Nixon. Daisy was only five years old when Harry Truman took office." Dr. Jennings gave Mama other memory tests and she failed all of them. Finally, Dr. Jennings concluded, "Daisy has Alzheimer's disease." There was a long silence. Daddy began to stutter, "What's next? What's the treatment for Alzheimer's?"

Based on her level of confusion, the symptoms Mama exhibited probably began many years before her actual diagnosis. Mama's memory lapses occurred without consistency, making it difficult to identify the problem, and thus we were not able to seek intervention that might have helped preserve her memory and slow the degeneration of her cognitive function.

Before we knew she had Alzheimer's, Mama had started putting sticky notes on things throughout the house. At first, I wrote it off as Mama's way of getting better organized. On one particular day, however, I paid Mama a surprise visit. I was shocked to find she had sticky notes on almost everything in the kitchen, including easily recognizable items that she had used all her life. She had sticky notes on all of her seasonings in the cabinet. There were notes on cabinet doors and notes on items stored in their normal place. She even wrote "salt" and "pepper" on sticky notes on the salt and pepper shakers! I finally questioned her about it, and she said, "I was just reorganizing the kitchen." We laughed about it, and I dropped the subject, telling myself not to worry because it was her house and her kitchen and she could do whatever she wanted with it. The next time I visited, I saw all the sticky notes were gone. Then I believed she knew I was on to her that something was wrong, and this might have been her way to try to throw me off the trail.

Mama always cooked a large meal on Sunday, and my family would come over and have dinner with my parents on a regular basis. One week, we all were in the dining room eating, and Mama asked me to get the cornbread out of the oven. I went to the kitchen to do as she asked, and to my surprise, the cornbread was not in the oven and the oven was not on. Then Mama asked me to get the sweet tea from the refrigerator while I was in the kitchen. When I opened the door to the refrigerator, I found the cornbread in there. On another Sunday, the cornbread made it to the oven, but Mama forgot to put eggs in the batter, so it came out flat. Sunday dinners began to taste more than interesting as time progressed. Mama would always make excuses for how the meal came out, such as, "I was trying a new recipe, so it may taste a little different." This was unusual in and of itself, as Mama was always an excellent cook who never second-guessed her recipes, old or new. When the outcome was not good, she would joke about it. Then one year, for her annual New Year's dinner, Mama burned much of the meal. This was her signature event each year, and she was expecting about forty people. She stopped cooking altogether shortly after that.

Another time Mama hemmed two pair of pants for me and the cuffs were six inches long instead of a traditional one to two inches. The symptoms of Alzheimer's became more frequent and more bizarre—and more unpredictable. In 2005, Mama had three car accidents, and each accident occurred when another driver ran into Mama's vehicle. Mama would not be specific with information, so no one pressed her for details. We continued to believe these were coincidences until Daddy finally came to the realization something was not quite right with Mama. Daddy stopped Mama from driving because she had three car accidents within a 12-month period each of accidents, the police ruled the other driver at fault. However, based on the signs she was exhibiting, there may have been more to these accidents. Daddy retired from General Motors, and I realized this was a major turning point for Mama and Daddy.

After Mama's diagnosis, I thought it might not be so bad. Mama's forgetfulness was sometimes humorous at first. But after a while, it was no longer amusing. Her behavior became even more unpredictable, and at times, violent. Mama's behavior was contrary to who she was before the diagnosis. As the disease progressed, Mama's episodes became longer and more frequent, and certainly more unlike her normal persona. Mama began using profanity and acted violently toward people she did not recognize. Her behavior was disturbing to members of our family because Mama had never used profanity or acted violently before.

Because Mama's ability to socialize was steadily declining, I began to witness how the Alzheimer's was changing each of her relationships. Prior to Mama's diagnosis, none of us had any experience with the disease. Perhaps this is one of the reasons none of us were able to recognize the symptoms. Her episodes were so inconsistent, and none of us suspected or wanted to believe it was attributed to such an awful disease. We all had to overcome our disbelief in our own way and in our own time. We all probably continue to work at it in some form or fashion.

I did not know what Alzheimer's really was, and I did not know what Alzheimer's symptoms looked like. I thought someone with Alzheimer's would simply occasionally forget the names of loved ones. I slowly began to realize that Alzheimer's would eventually rob Mama of all of her memories, including events she had participated in, relationships she had developed, knowledge she had acquired, and skills she had learned. Worse still, I came to understand that Alzheimer's would also rob Mama of the ability to create and maintain new memories. I hated to think and did not want to believe that Mama could have such an awful and incurable disease. Mama had had a long career as a teacher for St. Louis Public Schools. Mama had always been healthy and conscious of maintaining her well-being. She had been athletic, energetic, and usually on the go. As her disease progressed, Mama forgot how to cook, sew, and even how to comb her own hair.

Scripture Help: "About the ninth hour Jesus cried out in a loud voice...My God, my God, why have you forsaken me" (Matt. 27:46 NIV)? "Listen to my prayer, O God do not ignore my plea; hear me and answer me. My thoughts trouble me and I am distraught" (Ps. 55.1 NIV).

Prayer: Lord, the troubles, and disappointments are mounting. I want to go to sleep and wake up with the trouble and disappointment no longer there. I wake up and nothing has changed. Lord, continue to remind us that you did not promise a life with no suffering. You promised that you would be with us always, now and into eternity. Lord, I do not understand, why Alzheimer's? Why does this disease take away so many precious memories? Lord, I trust and believe you will be there when sufferers are alone with no memories. Lord, I trust and believe you will be there when caregivers are alone and tired. Lord, give us the wisdom and the strength to navigate through the disappointment and lead us through this incredible trial. Alzheimer's is a major turning point for sufferers and caregivers, yet our trust is in you. Lord, bless them with your grace and your mercy. In Jesus' holy name we pray. Amen.

Chapter 4:

It's a Family Affair

Family is conflict, and it's something that we all relate to.
—Bill Cosby

*J*ohnnie and Mary Phillips, my mother's parents, had eleven children who grew up in a tight-knit family in Winona, Mississippi. Mama had two sisters: Mae Judy of Grenada, Mississippi and Mary of St. Louis, Missouri. She had eight brothers: Jack of Memphis, Tennessee, B. F. of St. Louis, Missouri, and Lee Eddie, Edward, William (Bo), Howard, George, and Thomas of Winona, Mississippi. Mama was the sixth child born to Johnnie and Mary's union. The family was obviously large, as well as emotionally close. No significant event in any of Mama's siblings' lives ever went unnoticed, uncelebrated, unexamined, or unaddressed. An army of family members praised, prayed, persevered, organized, attended, participated, observed, or celebrated as each situation required. Even though I was nearly three hundred miles from Mama's roots in Mississippi, at many times I felt as though the family lived just around the corner. Mama was a teacher and the one benefit that teachers have is the time off. We were in Mississippi for nearly every holiday with the exception of New Year's. I spent every Christmas in Mississippi until I was married with children.

In late summer of 1985, Mama Mary's brother, Bud, had a stroke. The news was shocking to Mama Mary, who was alone at the time.

As a way of calming down and coping with the news of her dear brother, Mama Mary decided to lie down and see if she could rest before the rest of her family came home. When Mama Mary woke up from her nap, she had no memory of herself or anyone else, which caused her great distress. When Papa Johnnie came home and discovered her in an agitated condition, he did not know the reason for her dismay. He looked around the room and quickly went to his wife's side to console her, asking her what the matter was. She was starting to calm down, but he still decided to take her to the hospital.

The emergency doctors diagnosed her as having short-term temporary memory loss and confusion. They said such a condition was likely caused by the traumatic stress of receiving such bad news about her brother, Bud, with whom she was very close.

Mama heard about her mother's episode and immediately decided to visit her mother in Mississippi. Mama took my sister, Iris, and me along so we could perhaps cheer her up a bit. Mama Mary loved all of her grandchildren, and she seemed to light up whenever any of us were around, no matter how old we got. Mama did not explain many details to Iris and me on our way to Mississippi. She only said Mama Mary was tired and needed rest. Mama seemed pensive on this trip south, and she appeared to be a bit anxious and impatient about arriving.

After a hasty ride in the car in which we rarely stopped for gasoline or snacks, as we usually would have, we finally arrived in Winona. I spent most of the first day observing Mama Mary and her movements around the house, as well as other family members' reactions to what she was doing. Mama Mary seemed to be having amnesia-like symptoms. She recognized some family members easily, some she recognized with coaching and a bit of effort, and some she did not recognize at all. She also seemed to be able to manage some daily tasks, but she was unable to perform other simple things, such as cooking, bathing, and dressing. She appeared confused and annoyed at times; other times she was despondent and fearful. Papa Johnnie assumed the role of primary caregiver and did everything for her, even though he had an army of relatives willing and able to step in and help him. For most of the visit, relatives were ready to spring into action, but they were never called to serve, so the mood was quiet and somber. The visit was tense and unpredictable, unlike any visit we'd had in the past. Usually our times together were happy times, with easy-flowing conversation, laughter, and a great deal of activity.

I later realized that there are strong and undeniable parallels in the symptoms Mama Mary and my own Mama exhibited.

Some relatives believed Mama Mary must have had a stroke, which caused her memory loss and other peculiar behavior. Others wrote her behavior off to her getting a little older, being a little tired, or maybe working a little too hard around the house. A few family members did not offer any opinions. But we all worried the same.

I was so unused to this kind of talk in Winona. The can-do spirit of the family was always evident, and illnesses were viewed as mere annoyances that would never sabotage ultimate family goals. The network of family members here was so strong, so visible, and so available; I never once considered there was a weakness in the chain. This visit opened my eyes to the possibility that my family was vulnerable to things beyond our control. And for the first time, I took a hard look around the room and noticed that some family members were getting older, moved slower, and weren't as razor-sharp as I always assumed they would be. I began to see my family as they really were instead of as I remembered them and preferred to view them. When I looked at Mama, who was still pensive and anxious, for the first time I noticed she had aged, too.

Mama Mary did not live long after her September episode with amnesia. She died of congestive heart failure on February 13, 1986. In the days preceding her death, Mama Mary's memory seemed to improve. And in many respects, she went back to her old routines around the house. She was well enough to resume cooking, cleaning, and washing clothes, and she appeared happy and healthy. The family rejoiced at the power and grace of the Lord because he had removed her infirmity and restored her health to what seemed to be even better than before her episode.

After other family members reported the good news, Uncle Edward remained skeptical; he came to Mama Mary's house for a visit so he could see for himself how well Mama Mary had miraculously recovered. Uncle Edward marveled at her recovery and watched her every move intently, as if he were trying to verify the miracle. As he was watching her cook, Uncle Edward sat reminiscing about how life used to be before Mama Mary got ill, and he savored the memories of her wonderful cooking.

"Won't you stay for dinner?" Mama Mary said to Uncle Edward. He eagerly obliged the request, believing, yes, things were getting back to normal. As she dished the piping hot food from the stove onto serving platters, she hummed a little song that must have been repeating in her head. A smile came to her lips as she moved from the stove to the table, where her son was sitting and waiting for his first spoonful of the delicious dinner. They sat together and blessed the food, and then began to eat.

Yes, things are getting back to normal, Uncle Edward thought as he enjoyed the meal and his mother's company. The food, fantastic as usual, reminded him of better times from a long-ago era. He looked around at the kitchen and remembered each what-not on the shelves and walls. The crisp and fresh breeze blew gently through the back window and cooled his face. His mother's smile, evident and warm, was a permanent fixture amongst these memories.

But, oddly, her smile was not present now. He looked at his mother and took her hand, interrupting her thoughts as she negotiated her plate of food and gingerly took insufficient and laborious bites. Mama Mary then made a statement that drew the color from Uncle Edward's face. "This is the last meal I am ever going to eat with you," Mama Mary said to Uncle Edward.

Stunned, he stared at his plate of food, and then looked up to meet her gaze. She looked wistful as she chewed. They continued their meal in silence. After several long moments, Mama Mary said, "I am going to be dead in three days."

Uncle Edward responded quickly, anxious for an explanation. "What makes you think this?" Uncle Edward asked.

Mama Mary said, "Jesus told me. He said these last few months of my having spells was to help the family prepare for it. He told me the family is ready now."

Uncle Edward sat in utter disbelief, at a loss for words and unable to process what he had just heard. He pushed his plate away, no longer hungry, and rose from the table. Shoving his hands in his pockets, he paced the floor of the kitchen while Mama Mary sat in her place. Deciding he could do nothing else, he came back to the table and hugged her. The meal over, they sat in the kitchen and held hands while the sunset and the night air turned chilly.

When Uncle Edward returned home, he called his other siblings and told them what Mama Mary had said over dinner and described the evening he had shared with her. Mama Mary died three days later.

After Mama Mary's passing, we learned that Uncle Jack, Mama's eldest brother, had been diagnosed with Alzheimer's disease. At first, the family had believed that his mood swings, memory loss, and general disposition might have been because he was still grieving the loss of his wife, Margaret. After the diagnosis, the family realized his behavior was indicative of the moderate stages of Alzheimer's disease. Uncle Jack exhibited more and more signs of problems in his daily routine and activities, and less coordination, recall, and emotional control.

Because Uncle Jack lived in Memphis, I saw him only occasionally at family functions and special occasions, and thus did not know what his normal routine might have been. Admittedly, many of those initial signs would not have caught my notice, nor would many other members of the family have immediately realized there was a problem.

I became aware of a difference in Uncle Jack's behavior when I co-hosted a family reunion with my sister, Iris. The reunion took place in St. Louis, and one of our planned activities was a family outing to the St. Louis Zoo. While we were visiting the zoo, Uncle Jack separated from the group and became lost. We were not initially worried, believing he may have just found a shady spot to sit for a while or perhaps went in another direction to find the restroom. After more than thirty minutes of looking around in the general vicinity and not locating Uncle Jack, we became worried. At this point we stopped discounting the symptoms of confusion, agitation, and memory loss. Once he had gone missing for nearly an hour, we started putting some of the pieces together. Shortly after the family reunion, Uncle Jack was diagnosed with Alzheimer's, and the family understood and agreed with the diagnosis. Uncle Jack lived with Alzheimer's for several years and progressively declined during over time. Before passing away, Uncle Jack's condition declined to a vegetative state, and for awhile, he was on life support.

Many months after Mama's own diagnosis of Alzheimer's in 2008, Mama's oldest sister, Aunt Mae Judy, also began exhibiting symptoms of the disease. She was diagnosed in the moderate stages, bringing the number of diagnoses in the family to four. Each victim experienced significant memory impairment, confusion, agitation, and mood swings, all of which adversely affected their quality of life. None of my family members with the disease was able to do daily activities independently, nor could they make decisions for their own affairs, safety, health, wants, or needs.

Members of my family have discovered that learning a loved one has been afflicted with Alzheimer's is shocking, to say the least. We have all been apprehensive to accept the effects the disease has on those we love. And most of us have found ourselves in a state of denial, fear and uncertainty.

We have all asked ourselves these questions. How would one cope with this devastating fate? How, as a family, do we continue to move forward? How do we continue to honor, love, and care for the family members who suffer from the disease? How do the caregivers find the strength, encouragement, and resolve to continue to do what is vital to the health and well-being of the sufferer?

The family unit is the answer. Together, we celebrate the good times, and together, we endure the times of trial. What matters the most is we are in it together, getting through whatever we face in the days ahead.

Mama has always been about family. She believes all aspects of life are a family affair. For this reason, I do not see this as something she is suffering through alone, with her family on the sidelines. We are in this together with her, as well as with our other family members who suffer from the disease. Mama's touch transcends the disease. She was a significant part of our lives before her diagnosis, and her influence will continue to touch our lives long after the disease claims the last bit of her.

As I continued to reflect on Mama's life, I realized that in her heart was one constant. She lived by the words, "So that there should be no division in the body, but that its parts should have equal concern for each other. If one part suffers, every part suffers with it; if one part is honored, every part rejoices with it. Now you are the body of Christ, and each one of you is a part of it" (1 Cor. s 12:25-27 NIV). Since she taught me this truth over the years, it helped prepare me to face the challenges that confronted me as I helped care for her, and most of all, decided to tell our story.

Scripture Help: "So do not fear, for I am with you; do not be dismayed, for I am your God. I will strengthen you and help you; I will uphold you with my righteous right hand" (Isa. 41:10 NIV).

Prayer: Lord, thank you for all of the wonderful blessings you have provided. We lift up in prayer Alzheimer's suffers, caregivers and their families. This disease is hard on everyone. Ease their pain as Alzheimer's continue to rob and destroy their memories one by one. We are all thankful for those who have gone before us and that we look forward to seeing them again in heaven. We rejoice in our ancestors' and family members' stories. We also rejoice in the ways the Lord makes his presence known in our lives through those who share their experience of Him with us. Lord, you are awesome! In Jesus' name, I pray. Amen.

Chapter 5:

Death at a Funeral

Don't be afraid to feel as angry or as loving as you can,
because when you feel nothing, it's just death.
—Lena Horne

Mama's oldest brother, Jack, passed away from Alzheimer's. Uncle Jack was Mama's first sibling to have passed away since her diagnosis of Alzheimer's. Uncle Jack was Mama's eldest sibling, who lived in Memphis, Tennessee. During Uncle Jack's funeral, Mama seemed to be doing well. After the funeral, the pall-bearers carried Uncle Jack's casket to the hearse, and family and friends began to socialize and comfort one another.

It appeared Mama was still doing okay; unfortunately, Mama was not doing well. Suddenly, Mama frantically began asking who died. I responded, "Your brother, Jack." After becoming upset, she cried out with a painful tremble in her voice, "Why didn't anyone tell me Jack had died?" Mama became upset and angry; it was horrifying. Mama asked again and again, "Who died?" In Mama's mind, Jack's death was recurring repeatedly at the funeral. Next, Mama asked to see Jack's body; the funeral directors were kind and honored Mama's request. They rolled the casket out of the hearse and let her view the body one last time. The last viewing of Uncle Jack's body seemed to give Mama the closure she needed. To watch Mama go through this level of recurring grief and anguish was heart-wrenching. After the experience, we knew this would be the last funeral Mama would ever attend.

Uncle Jack was a great role model for all of his sisters and brothers. Nevertheless, his death brought Mama deep sadness. Mama's fragmented memory did not allow her to retain the knowledge that Uncle Jack had died. She continued to relive the sad news of his death over and over again as if it were the very first time she had heard about it, so she was unable to properly grieve his death. I felt the vibrations of her agony. Mama's grief was as if her heart suffered multiple stab wounds with no knowledge of the previous wound. Each time she learned of his death, it seemed to occur in slow motion, allowing her to intensely see and feel every second of this moment. Daddy held her closer and tighter each time her knees became weak from hearing the painful news, "Uncle Jack has died."

The pain and grief of my Uncle Jack's death brought back the heartache we felt when my grandmother, Mama Mary, died in 1986. At my grandmother's funeral, I stood with Mama as we watched the funeral directors cover the casket with dirt. Each scoop of the shovel was amplified, and the thump from the dirt falling on the casket felt so final. I think Mama and I both went into a trance; each shovel of dirt represented letting go. I believe we both felt as though we were passing with each thump of dirt like a fading heart-beat. The sound of dirt falling became more and more faint, and I saw Mama become more and more lifeless. I hoped someone would call her name, call my name. We both were sinking. I wanted someone to touch Mama so we both could let go and move on. I will never forget that painful memory.

As Mama's Alzheimer's progressed, in her mind deceased relatives were still alive. It seemed like Mama's brain was deleting all of her painful memories and keeping only the good memories. Perhaps forgetting the death of family members may be one of the few benefits of having Alzheimer's disease. To the sufferer, everyone lives forever.

Scripture Help: "The righteous cry out, and the LORD hears them; he delivers them from all their troubles. The LORD is close to the brokenhearted and saves those who are crushed in spirit" (Ps. 34:17–18

NIV). God can bring comfort to us when we have suffered a loss of someone dear to us.

Prayer: I thank you, Lord, for being my strength when I was weak. God help me to know joy and seek joy in those times of intense sadness. In my joy, I can find divine strength and refuge. Your amazing peace allows me to be joyful and sad at the same time. Lord, you are the almighty God I seek. My relationship with you is my greatest treasure. I thank you for the strength you continue to give Alzheimer's sufferers and their caregivers as the disease progresses. Lord, we thank you for the joy to smile. Thank you for the serenity we regularly see on their face. Lord, please continue to bless each of us with joy as the Alzheimer's disease progresses. Lord, continue to bless us all with strength, courage, and wisdom to exhibit your love, peace and kindness. Thank you, Lord, for allowing Alzheimer's sufferers and caregivers to know you are with them in both the highs and the lows of life. I ask all of these things in the name of your dearest Son, Jesus. Amen.

Chapter 6:

Stranger in My House

Like any artist without an art form, she became dangerous.
—Toni Morrison

 was home doing my chores and my phone rang. It was Daddy. He said my name, and immediately I knew something was not right. I asked, "Is everything OK?" He paused and then replied, "I am okay, but Daisy has been fighting me!" I replied, "I am on my way!"

This trip to my parents' house seemed to take longer than it ever had before. After pulling up in the driveway, I saw Daddy sitting in a lawn chair in the garage with the cordless phone in his hand. Daddy's eyes were red, and I could tell he had been crying. I said, "Daddy, what is going on?" He explained to me that Mama had been hitting him with a broom, and she didn't know who he was.

I took a deep breath and quietly said a quick prayer. I entered the house from the garage and immediately scanned the kitchen, family room, dining room, and living room for any signs of Mama. I continued down the hallway and found Mama lying down on the bed in my old room; she was wide-awake underneath a pile of clothes and rubbing her feet together. Mama and I both have this habit of rubbing our feet together when we are lying down, either relaxing or thinking.

I asked, "Mama, what are you doing?" Her response was, "Nothing." I replied, "Mama, I hear you have been fighting!" Mama stood up and walked out of the bedroom, down the hallway, and to the living room. She told her version of the story as she walked around the living room using her hands; she began to tell me an incredible story about a man who had broken into the house and was touching her. She asked him to leave, and he would not. Mama called the police, and the police came and arrested the strange man. Meanwhile, she got her broom and beat the man up and knocked him down; then the police came and arrested the man.

I continued with my investigation, "So, Mama, what did the strange man look like?" Mama replied, "He was young and light-skinned!" Daddy then came into the room, and I asked Mama, "Is this the man who was bothering you?" Mama replied, "No, that is an old man! The man they arrested was young and light-skinned." I asked her, "Mama, who is this old man?" Mama paused as though she was thinking and replied, "I don't know!" I said, "Mama, do you know who I am?" Mama replied, "I know who you are. You are Junior."

Mama became frustrated and she offered me several iterations of the story, and each time the story became more and more elaborate. Before she told the story each time, she paused and asked where my daddy, Norris, was. Daddy continued to stand in the room with his hands clasped together, hoping and anticipating that she escape this loop of confusion she was in. Then she finally looked at him with a long stare and suddenly recognized who he was. Daddy smiled and Mama smiled. She demanded to know, "Norris, where have you been? I have been looking for you. Remember, you are not supposed to leave me." Mama open her arms and walked toward Daddy and they both embraced each other and they walked into the living room holding hands and sat down next to each other on the couch.

God's Word says, "Have I not commanded you? Be strong and courageous. Do not be terrified; do not be discouraged, for the LORD your God will be with you wherever you go" (Josh. 1:9 NIV). The one thing Mama did not lack was courage; only Daddy and I were terrified. I admired Mama's courage in this moment in spite of her condition; Mama was not the least bit discouraged or scared. I found her lying on my old bed with a small collection of her clothes draped across her, simply relaxing. This was not the first time I had to come over help my parents through a spell like this. I believe what made this situation different was that I had prayed to God for courage, strength, and wisdom.

In Mama's confusion, Daddy went from being twenty years old to sixty-nine in just a few hours; yet in her mind, everything was OK. Daddy shrugged it off and said, "This is part of Alzheimer's, and together we will get through it."

"Until now you have not asked for anything in my name. Ask and you will receive, and your joy will be complete" (John 16:24 NIV). In this very moment, I saw the strength of my parents and a glimpse of the bond they continue to share. I thank you, Lord, for answering my prayers so quickly.

Scripture Help: "Two are better than one, because they have a good return for their work: If one falls down, his friend can help him up! Also, if two lie down together, they will keep warm. But how can one keep warm alone? Though one may be overpowered, two can defend themselves. A cord of three strands is not quickly broken" (Eccles. 4:9–12 NIV).

Prayer: Lord, I bring before you all Alzheimer's sufferers and care-givers. Alzheimer's disease profoundly affects their lives. When they feel diminished, remind them that you know their suffering, and you call them by name. Lord, you hold them and every situation in the palm of your hand. Help to us to know that you are always near when we feel fragile and broken. Lord, we thank you for healing and molding us into Christ's image as we continue to face the challenges of Alzheimer's disease. Lord, when we feel uncertain about our future, lead us to your perfect love and your perfect peace. Your love casts out all fear and doubt. Lord, when situations and circumstances make us think we cannot go on, remind us, "love never fails, and, living in your love; they will bear your fruit in plenty" (1 Cor. 13:8 NIV). Lord, help our families to have the courage always to love each other in every situation. Lord, thank you for hearing our prayers. In Jesus' darling name I pray. Amen.

Chapter 7:

Before I Let Go

Some think it's holding on that makes one strong;
sometimes it's letting go.
—Sylvia Robinson

*E*ight months after Mama's diagnosis of Alzheimer's disease, it became clear to Mama and Daddy that she was not going to be able to make those long trips to Mississippi anymore. The symptoms were progressing quickly and her wandering was increasing. The advancement of her disease was a big game-changer for how we could interact and care for Mama. Mama would do the best she could to pretend that she did not have Alzheimer's, and we all cooperated with her. We thought if we acted as if everything was normal, she would be normal. Sometimes we were all able to fool ourselves, yet the disease continued to progress, even though Mama was undergoing treatment. And unfortunately, her disease was evolving faster than even the doctors had projected.

According to the Alzheimer's Association, six in ten people with Alzheimer's wander, which means they become disoriented in familiar places, such as their home or places they had often frequented (2012). In Mama's case, she would try or would want to "go home," even when she was already at home. Mama also had difficulty locating familiar places in her home such as the bathroom, the bedroom, or the kitchen. Daddy got especially upset when Mama would get out-of-sorts and ask the whereabouts of someone who was sitting right next to her. The wandering behavior sometimes coupled with restlessness; she would often pace throughout the house with repetitive movements.

Mama and Daddy decided to make one last trip to Mississippi while Mama still had enough memory to make the trip without difficulty. Fall of 2009, Mama and Daddy asked my sister and me to join them for this last trip with our families to Mississippi. This trip was different for many reasons. Mama's father, Papa Johnnie, was no longer living in the home where Mama grew up; he was in a nursing home. Usually we would lodge at Mama's childhood home on New Hope Road in Winona, Mississippi, but this time we all lodged together at a hotel in Grenada, Mississippi. This trip was also different because we did not go from house to house to visit family. Family came to us at the hotel where we were staying for fellowship.

Transitions, or moving from one place or activity to another, were becoming more and more difficult for Mama. We found that the easiest way to get her through transitions was to use speed and patience. In the case of moving from the house to the car, I would sometimes simply pick Mama up and carry her to the car as fast as I could. Before she had time to respond aggressively or negatively, I would have her buckled in her seat.

After we checked into the hotel in Grenada, Mississippi, we called the family to let them know we had arrived. We decided to stay in the hotel and not with relatives to avoid any unnecessary transitions for Mama. We arrived late in the evening, and we had dinner at the "Fish House" with my Uncle Howard, his wife Aunt Shirley, and my Uncle Albert, Daddy's brother. Mama did not exhibit any of her common symptoms. After dinner, we met with Aunt Mae Judy, Mama's oldest sister, and a few of my first cousins in the hotel room. Mama was talkative and funny. She had many of us in stitches, laughing. It was so good to see her not having a memory lapse while visiting with her sister. Mama was doing so well, Mama and Daddy continued with their plans to visit Papa Johnnie at the nursing home for the whole next day. Aunt Mae Judy called our other relatives to let them know she wanted everyone to be at the nursing home the next day with Daisy and her family.

It was amazing to see Mama with Papa Johnnie. While we were visiting at the nursing home, Mama did not exhibit any Alzheimer's symptoms. This was an incredible blessing, and Mama very much wanted it to happen this way. Many relatives visited while we were at the nursing home. It was like old times; Mama's presence once again brought everyone together. This was the last time we all were together before Papa Johnnie passed away.

I believe Mama wanted to create one more moment for all of us before she had to let go. The Alzheimer's was progressing quickly, and she wanted to create one last memory for us to cherish before she progressed to a stage when this memory would not be possible. Bringing everyone together was one of Mama's many gifts. Because of Mama, we had another wonderful memory that we would always cherish. The one thing I never factored into life was that things change. With age comes fading health. As we age, our bodies cannot continue to do the things it once did before. Mama was one of the healthiest people I was in close contact with. Yet she was not exempt from Alzheimer's disease, which would wither her mind. Alzheimer's was so overwhelming I found myself losing heart.

Scripture Help: "Therefore we do not lose heart. Though outwardly we are wasting away, yet inwardly we are being renewed day by day. For our light and momentary troubles are achieving for us an eternal glory that far outweighs them all. So we fix our eyes not on what is seen, but on what is unseen. For what is seen is temporary, but what is unseen is eternal" (2 Cor. 4:16–18 NIV).

Prayer: Lord, bless Alzheimer's sufferers and allow them to fulfill their last wishes while they have enough memory left to share their hearts before letting go. Lord, we thank you for your strength. Father, your love for us is boundless. May all members of each family love and respect each other, recognizing that we are all your children. Help us extend this love and respect to people outside our own families so you may be glorified. We pray that the standard of a godly family is restored. The moments of beauty in our lives is manifested in the likeness of God's beauty in the world through love for family. Lord, give us all the passion for family and the passion for fellowship. I thank you, Lord, for all the wonderful examples of family you deliver as we continue to journey through with Alzheimer's disease. In Jesus name I pray, Amen.

Chapter 8:

911 Emergency

Adrenaline is wonderful. It covers pain. It covers dementia.
It covers everything.
— Jerry Lewis

It was a beautiful, sunny day in St. Louis, and Daddy decided to take Mama for a drive. On the way back, they decided to get a carryout lunch from Captain D's. Daddy never used drive-through, even though he was going to order carryout. After getting back in the car, Daddy's speech became slurred, and he began to go in and out of consciousness. Somehow, Mama understood what was happening with Daddy; she knew he was in trouble. Mama got Daddy in the car on the passenger side and drove the SUV to their house. It must have been a divine adrenaline rush that enabled Mama to do what seemed impossible in her current condition. Mama drove home, entered into the house through garage, and called her sister, Aunt Mary Ann. Aunt Mary Ann called 911, and then she called me. Because I worked only a few minutes away, I arrived at my parents' house at the same time as the ambulance. I took a deep breath and whispered a prayer asking God for strength and mercy as I followed the paramedics into the house. My Aunt Mary Ann was standing at the front door beckoning the paramedics to come in with sense of urgency expressed on her face. Daddy was sitting in the chair in the living room next to front door and Mama was pacing the living room blanketed with worry and concern. Daddy was sweaty, shaky, and confused.

Aunt Mary Ann was obviously upset. However, as the two paramedics entered the front door, she calmly stated, "This is my brother-in-law and he is diabetic, exhibiting signs of low blood sugar." The male paramedic immediately measured Daddy's sugar levels while the female paramedic assessed his vitals. Mama was rubbing her hands nervously and whenever either of the paramedics asked Daddy a question, she would respond on his behalf. The male paramedics were recording Mama's responses on the wireless tablet. Moments later, a white male police officer showed up at the front door and entered the house. The officer introduced himself and began interviewing each of us. To my surprise, Mama was able to answer all his questions without any help. Mama responded with confidence and poise. Aunt Mary Ann and I were simply shocked with how well Mama was functioning in her condition.

Meanwhile, the paramedics measured Daddy's sugar levels. His sugar levels were dangerously low. Immediately, the female paramedic gave Daddy a sugar shot to shoot his sugar levels up. This was the first time Daddy had a low blood sugar episode. My wife, Jeannie, came through the open front door as we all greeted her with smiles. She returned a smile and asked, "So what is going on?" After Daddy's sugar levels measured at a normal state, the female paramedic said, "Mr. Roberts needs to eat a meal high in carbohydrates to sustain his sugar levels." Jeannie went into the kitchen and heated Daddy's "Captain D's dinner" in the microwave and brought it to him in the living room. I stayed close to Mama, ensuring that he would be okay. Daddy began to eat and we all started to relax. Daddy had stopped sweating and shaking.

The paramedic offered to take Daddy to the hospital, but he decided not to and signed the release form. The paramedics went on their way. After Daddy seemed to be ok, we focused our attention on Mama. Amazingly, Mama had come back to who she was before Alzheimer's in this brief time. After learning that Daddy was ok, she was happy and bursting with energy; not like before when the paramedics and the rest of us were taking care of Daddy. As I reflected on what had just happened, Mama seemed confident and unshakable, and she began to explain what had happened. All I could say was, "Look at God go!" It seemed incredible that Mama was her old self, and I rejoiced in her renewed capacity. The absence of symptoms from Mama's disease for this brief period was a miracle.

At the time of the incident with Daddy, Mama had not driven a vehicle in more than two years; she had been unable to recall her own address, telephone number, or the name of the high school or college from which she graduated. At this stage of the disease, Mama was often confused about where she was or what day it was. She also needed help dressing herself and had begun to wander; she would sometimes attempt to leave the house alone to find her parents.

After the 911 emergency was over, and the adrenaline had subsided, I sat on the couch next to Mama. She sat on the living room couch with her legs crossed, and she smiled and held my hand. This moment reminded me of the time when my daughter, JJ, was involved in a nearly fatal go-kart accident at Winners Pointe near my residence in Saint Peters. Since Mama's diagnosis of Alzheimer's, I often find myself reflecting on our reactions during other times of stress to help me cope with the losses of Alzheimer's.

JJ's accident occurred on a breezy spring day. I thought it was the perfect day to do something unscheduled and fun with the twins, but unfortunately, despite the perfection of the day, we suffered a very scary freak accident. While she was driving around the track for fun, suddenly, all of the safety features on the go-kart failed, and JJ lost control. The go-kart jumped track barriers, sped across the parking lot, and crashed into a chain-link fence. The go-kart pedal was stuck, and the top rail of the chain-link fence caught JJ's neck. It took me and two other men to hold the go-kart in place until one of the workers figured out a way to disable the go-kart. If we had not intervened, the pressure from the fence could have broken her neck. Once the pedal was disengaged, we were able to remove her from the go-kart. Fortunately, she only suffered head, face, and neck injuries; she was OK for the most part. My emotions felt like they had separated into a thousand pieces. My wife, Jeannie, was out of town in Chicago on our church's women's mission trip, and I was alone in the hospital with my injured daughter and son. Cell phones were not yet popular. Fortunately, Mama was home to receive my call.

After I called Mama to let her know what had happened, I realized that I had forgotten to tell her we were at Barnes Saint Peter's Hospital. I called Mama back to let her know the name of the hospital, but she had already left. I contacted the nurse and told her I forgot to tell my mother the name of the hospital and location. I asked the nurse to call St. Joseph Hospital to let the emergency staff know where Mama should go if she went there to look for us.

But amazingly, Mama had already hurried to the hospital emergency room where we were. Mama did this with no help or instruction from hospital staff, and she bypassed all security doors and staff. Mama always was able to sense the whereabouts of her children, even when I was little.

Mama's display of courage and strength after Daddy's spell reminded me of how blessed we were throughout our lives. Despite her Alzheimer's, Mama continued to display amazing strength, will, and determination in the most extreme circumstances.

Scripture Help: "I lift up my eyes to the hills—where does my help come from? My help comes from the LORD, the Maker of heaven and earth. He will not let your foot slip—he who watches over you will not slumber; indeed, he who watches over Israel will neither slumber nor sleep. The LORD watches over you—the LORD is your shade at your right hand; the sun will not harm you by day, nor the moon by night. The LORD will keep you from all harm—he will watch over your life; the LORD will watch over your coming and going both now and forevermore" (Ps. 121:1-8 NIV).

Prayer: Lord, we thank you for your loving kindness and we thank you for your watchful eye. No matter what the problem, storm or trial, you have the answer and graciously send help to our rescue. I thank you, Lord, for your protection. Lord, I thank you for seeing our emergencies and dispatching help and comfort in miraculous ways. Your help gives each of us a testimony of your continuous love and devotion. In Jesus' name, I pray. Amen.

Chapter 9:

You Belong to Me

We do not remember days, we remember moments.
The richness of life lies in memories we have forgotten.
—Cesare Pavese

*I*t was an unusually warm and beautiful day in Saint Louis. I was running errands and decided to drop in on my parents to see how they were doing. I rang the doorbell and there was no answer, so I let myself in. I called for Mama and Daddy with a cheerful hello; something that seemed to complement the day's sunny weather. Daddy answered, "We are in the bedroom." As I proceeded toward their room, I heard them laughing and listening to music.

As I got to the doorway, Daddy spoke gently to Mama and said, "Daisy, who is that?" She gave me a long stare and said, "I don't know who you are, but I know you belong to me, and you look good to me." Mama was smiling and laughing, and she reached out to give me hug. This was such a wonderful greeting from Mama, given all we had recently endured with her condition. Daddy chirped, "Daisy, it is your son, Junior." Mama threw her hands up in the air and replied, "Come here, sweetheart, and let me get a good look at you! You sure are handsome, and I know you belong to me; I can't recall your name, but it is okay!" For the moment, it did not bother me that she could not recall my name; what mattered was she knew I was no stranger to her. What mattered was she knew I was someone she loved and cared for. It made the greeting memorable and the moment quite wonderful.

I savored this moment with my parents. It was a healing moment, I believed, for all three of us. Perhaps this was another turning point. What if Mama could not remember my name ever again, or forgot I was someone she loved and cared for? What would happen on the day she no longer recognized those facts? I decided not to focus on negative thoughts. What was important and most significant was that Mama knew my spirit.

At this stage, Mama still had conversations, but she was occasionally exhibiting symptoms of paranoia and aggression. She was also beginning to lose weight because she was not eating. Sometimes she did not remember to eat, and other times her brain would tell her she was not hungry, which was a common characteristic of Alzheimer's patients.

She was also going through a phase of putting on multiple outfits at the same time. Sometimes when I would see her, I thought about my grandparents' scarecrows in the fields in Mississippi. The fragmented nature of my memories felt funny to me. I thanked God for the memories he allowed me to retrieve, even when they came in bits and pieces.

As her Alzheimer's progressed, Mama's spiritual sense seemed to be heightening. I perceived that Mama's spirit was compensating for her mind, where this horrible disease had taken up unauthorized residence. With each passing day, the disease weakened Mama's body, yet her spirit appeared strengthened.

God showed me how to connect and communicate with Mama's spirit—the part of Mama that would eventually leave the earth to be with the Lord. At times we simply lay on her bed together, holding hands, eyes closed—resting, communing, and finding fellowship in the spirit. Through this, she spiritually told me all the things she could not tell me physically, and I understood.

Lord, I came to realize that it was OK Mama could not remember my name and could no longer recall memories we shared together. It was so hard to let go of the way we were. When I gazed at Mama, I would recall when she was full of life and love. I wished for her to have good days, and I prayed for my strength and the strength of my family to help her through the not-so-good times.

Scripture Help: The Bible clearly establishes the fact that man is a triune being composed of spirit, soul, and body: "I pray God your whole spirit and soul and body be preserved blameless unto the coming of our Lord Jesus Christ" (1 Thess. 5:23 NIV). "For the word of God is quick, and powerful, and sharper than any two-edged sword, piercing even to the dividing asunder of soul and spirit, and of the joints and marrow (body), and is a discerner of the thoughts and intents of the heart" (Heb. 4:12 NIV).

Prayer: Lord, it becomes increasingly more difficult to stay close when the Alzheimer's sufferer's memories continue to fade. Lord, it seems so unfair how the losses continue to add up as the disease progresses. Lord, it seems that treasured memories are splintered and affections are battered. Lord, help me not to be angry, bitter or sad. Lord, I see that I am learning and growing on my journey with Alzheimer's disease. I am learning to trust you in minuscule ways. The suffering endured has evolved into a wonderful testimony of faith. Lord, I come to realize you are the one constant I have in this journey, and without you, it would be impossible to survive. I thank you for those times when I reminisce in a memory that makes me smile or laugh. Lord, the sweet memories seem to heal disappointments and remind me of how you have blessed me. Knowing you as my savior is my greatest blessing. Lord, use my journey as testimony to encourage caregivers and Alzheimer sufferers to look to you for their joy and peace. The joy that comes from you is their strength. And Lord, help them to keep holding on and never let go of your never-changing hand. In Jesus' name, I pray. Amen.

Chapter 10:

Anniversary

The heart of marriage is memories; and if the two of you
happen to have the same ones and can savor your reruns,
then your marriage is a gift from the gods.
—Bill Cosby

*S*torytelling was one of the earliest forms of human communication and learning. Mama's dementia prohibited her from being the storyteller, so I now took on the job. According to Silberner, storytelling could be therapeutic for those with dementia (2012). Telling narratives allowed Mama to be an active participant in a conversation. Mama was progressing into another chapter of Alzheimer's disease; she was not eating and had lost significant weight. Mama was so small I would lovingly say, "Mama, you got to eat something. We can't have you going back to high school skinny." Mama would laugh or begin her Naomi Campbell catwalk on her imaginary fashion runway. This would make us both laugh.

On Mama and Daddy's wedding anniversary, I wanted to bring them some chocolate-covered strawberries and a commemorative card. After I entered the house, I saw a bouquet of flowers on top of the china cabinet in the dining room. I thought this was a strange place for flowers. I made my way to the family room and saw Mama and Daddy sitting down together watching television. Daddy asked, "What do you have here?" I replied, "Chocolate-covered strawberries and a card." Daddy replied gladly, "Thank you! Thank you!" Daddy led me into the dining room and whispered, "Don't move those flowers. I gave Daisy those flowers, and she put the flowers in her mouth. She was trying to eat the roses. I will be damned; this shit is something else. It was a good call bringing her something she can eat. Daisy puts everything in her mouth; it is like she is a little kid again!" I was speechless and amazed.

Daddy said, "I am going to Cracker Barrel to get some dinner. What do you want?" I replied, "I will have the chicken and dumplings, carrots, and fried apples." I went back into the family room where Mama was sitting. I greeted her with a smile and a kiss on the forehead and sat down next to her. She reached over and took my hand. I began to remember stories she had shared about her brief courtship with Daddy and their wedding. I thought I would tell Mama their story. I became the storyteller. And I shared Mama's story with her once again.

On June 21, 1964, Mama married Norris Lee Roberts Sr. from Vaiden, Mississippi. Vaiden was an extremely small and rural town known for farming, and was approximately eleven miles south of Winona. Daddy was a handsome college-educated man who lived on a farm with his family and intended to farm as a career after taking a wife. A country boy at heart, he set his mind to finding a country girl who could share his interests as well as his values and his faith.

Daddy met Mama in downtown Winona. He was standing on the sidewalk shooting the breeze with a couple of his friends when suddenly he saw a gorgeous woman with an alluring walk. He checked her out from head-to-toe while removing his shades to get a better look. She walked by him. And as he stepped closer for a better look, he lost his balance and landed on his butt on the sidewalk.

Mama thought, *Mission accomplished!* Mama had a walk that could stop traffic, and she knew it. Mama walked over to him to introduce herself and extend her hand to help him up. Even though they had just met, Daddy immediately knew he had found the love of his life.

It was not easy for Daddy to court Mama. His many brothers and sisters demanded that he treat her with the utmost respect. Daddy found it easy to get along with her brothers and sisters and seemed to fit in right away. Her family's acceptance of him was a relief to Mama, who wanted everyone to admire him as she did.

The wedding took place on June 21, the first day of summer, in the front yard of Mama's family farm in Winona. Mama meticulously planned every detail of the wedding. She had dreamed of the perfect wedding since childhood. Mama was a visionary. She wanted to walk down the aisle, and since the farm had none, she created one herself from red brick pavers she placed in the center of the yard leading up to the porch. She also wanted to marry on the first day of summer. She believed it would symbolize the union was young, energetic, and with many days ahead.

On her wedding day, Mama stood 5 feet 3 inches tall, weighed 102 pounds, and measured 36-20-36. For a wedding gown, Mama's only available choice was to create a Daisy original, which would accommodate her curvaceous yet petite figure. The wedding dress was a short white ball gown with embroidered fabric and tulle. It fit Mama like a glove, and she was a vision of loveliness.

The dress only lasted about six years. In 1970, Mama ripped the dress apart and made my sister, Iris, an Easter dress with the fabric. Mama thought the fabric was too pretty to let it go to waste. She decided she wanted her daughter to have something special from her for a special day.

On their sunny and bright wedding day, the fragrance of flowers filled the air. Family came from everywhere, ready to embrace the enlarged clan and celebrate the union, which seemed to be blessed. During the ceremony, the parents of the bride and groom sat on the front porch while the rest of the family and friends stood on each side of the brick-paved aisle.

After the wedding, the two moved immediately to Daddy's family farm in Vaiden and settled in as husband and wife. Daddy's plan was to earn a living by farming the 150 acres of land. But Daddy and his father, Papa Anderson, could not agree on a fair financial arrangement. This led Mama and Daddy to do something unusual, to say the least, for both of them. They left Mississippi and found a new home in St. Louis. Since both of them were college educated and there was huge migration from southern states like Mississippi to cities like St. Louis and Chicago, they believed there would be many employment opportunities and an opportunity to build a home and a family together. Along with these plans, something else came along: me. Shortly after their marriage, I was conceived. So much of their planning now had to include how this move would take place with a growing family.

After Mama and Daddy made their decision to leave Mississippi, they decided Daddy would go to St. Louis to look for a job and find a place to live while Mama went back to Winona to live with her parents and have their baby. On March 1, 1965, Mama gave birth to her son, Norris Lee Roberts Jr., at Winona Hospital in Winona. Mama wanted her first child to be boy, and God answered her prayer. Mama used to tell me that, from the start, she and I shared a spiritual bond. She felt we could communicate without words. Our communication seemed to be of love in the purest form—unconditional, everlasting, and very deep.

Two months after I was born, Mama took a long train ride to join Daddy in St. Louis. She gathered our belongings, bundled her newborn in warm blankets, and set off on her adventure. I believe this moment was both very difficult and exciting for Mama. Moving to St. Louis was a very brave move for both Mama and Daddy. Neither of them had ever traveled outside of the state of Mississippi or lived more than fifty miles from home. Even though a state line and nearly three hundred fifty miles separated her, Mama was determined to stay connected with her parents and family. She made frequent trips, wrote letters, and called regularly, but she also remained connected through carrying on the cooking and other traditions she had learned over the years.

On my birthday for years, Mama would tell the story of how we first came to St. Louis. Mama would tell me, "I came to St. Louis on a train from Winona with you when you were only two months old, and you slept the entire way on a pillow on my lap." There were several train trips after that initial one. She loved to tell one story about a trip to Mississippi when I was a young boy. The train was quiet, and many people were napping. I was looking out the window, and I yelled out to Mama, "Mama, look! Look at all those horses!" The other passengers looked in the direction where I was pointing and discovered that I was actually looking at a pasture of cows. An amazing outburst of laughter followed. Mama said some people laughed so hard they had tears in their eyes! One of the passengers told Mama she needed to teach the baby the difference between a horse and a cow.

Without any doubt, there were significantly more opportunities in St. Louis than Mississippi for blacks in 1965. Daddy began his automotive career at General Motors, from where he eventually retired forty-two years later. And Mama began her teaching career at the St. Louis Public School System, from where she also retired forty-two years later. Mama often talked about how she passed her state teaching exam on the first attempt and how proud she was of this accomplishment. At the time, teachers could get a lifetime teaching certification, and Mama earned hers on her first attempt.

Scripture Help: "Love is patient, love is kind. It does not envy, it does not boast, it is not proud. It is not rude, it is not self-seeking, it is not easily angered, it keeps no record of wrongs. Love does not delight in evil but rejoices with the truth. It always protects, always trusts, always hopes, always perseveres" (1 Cor. 13: 4–7 NIV).

Prayer: Lord, I pray for all married couples that are struggling with Alzheimer's. Lord, all good things come from you and we thank you for the love and devotion you have implanted in the hearts of married couples that have continued the course of marriage for worst due to Alzheimer's. Lord, bless their union and help it to remain unshakable and unswerving through the Alzheimer's journey. Use their marriage to exhibit your patience, kindness, and commitment you have to all of us. Strengthen their faith to trust in you, and may your prudence guide their lives. Lord, bless all marriages with your peace and happiness. Continue to make their love fruitful for your glory. In Jesus' wonderful name, we pray. Amen.

Chapter 11:

Lost without You

The way to love anything is to realize that it may be lost.
— Gilbert K. Chesterton

$\mathcal{I}$t is spring of 2009. Mama's Alzheimer's had progressed to a point where Mama had really become a handful for Daddy. Mama was exhibiting more of the symptoms, such as wandering, agitation, paranoia, and not eating. Doctors and other healthcare professionals encouraged Daddy to use adult day care services. Mama and Daddy had always been private people, and Daddy wanted to continue to manage Mama's care privately, regardless of how difficult it became for him. I often wondered why he was so reluctant to get professional help. Was it stubbornness or simply a lack of trust?

I came to learn it was really a lack of trust. Daddy did not trust just anyone with Mama and he had good reason. Mama is his wife and Daddy accepted ultimate responsibility regardless of whose care she was in. That is his decision and Daddy owned that decision and took it seriously. Daddy also believed not everyone was equipped in handling Mama. Particularly, when she was experiencing an assaultive or violent episode and that included the professionals. And for the most part, Daddy's intuition was on point. After much thought and prayer, Daddy finally agreed to use the day care service for Mama. The adult day care provided a much-needed break for Daddy, who had been providing round-the-clock care for Mama. It was important for Mama to get specialized help with her cognitive and social stimulation, which could help slow the progression of her Alzheimer's.

Initially, Mama loved going to the adult day care facility. She would patiently wait for the van every day to pick her up and would get into the van without any problems. At the day care, Mama would do crafts and other activities and would often refer to the activities as classes she was taking. For many months, it was a great relief for Daddy and a great social outlet for Mama.

Unfortunately, after many months using adult day care services, Mama began to have problems there. Mama became socially withdrawn and her behavior became disruptive at the facility. Some of her behaviors included throwing food, hitting, and attempting to escape. Mama often got into trouble at the adult day care and would frequently be sent home. This was frustrating for Daddy. He would make plans to work in a community garden, walk, or spend time with his brother or cousins, but he would have to stop what he was doing and get Mama from the adult day care facility.

Once, during a game of bingo, Mama became agitated and gave one of the other female clients a black eye. After this incident, Daddy decided to decrease the use of the day care services from five days to two days a week. This change in her schedule seemed to work.

Then one day in the spring, Mama went to the bathroom, and after using the restroom, she slipped past the staff and left the building. Daddy received the call from the adult day care reporting that Mama was missing and had last been seen in the restroom. Officials of the organization contacted the local police department to help search for Mama. The local police identified that the adult day care had no wandering safeguards in place. Research states that only 31.3 percent of individuals with dementia or Alzheimer's who wander outside are found alive, and the cause of death is usually due to exposure, drowning, or being struck by a vehicle (Rowe, 2011). Daddy knew these facts, and he was worried sick; all he wanted was to find Mama alive and well. To my surprise, Daddy did not call my sister, Iris, my aunt Mary Ann, or me. He stayed near the phone at home and just prayed, asking God not to let Mama's life end this way. He always wanted Mama to die peacefully and with dignity; that is very important to him. Daddy prayed for Mama's safe return.

Mama was missing for five hours. She was eventually found wandering miles away from the adult day care in a retired schoolteacher's backyard. The retired teacher spotted Mama from her kitchen window and knew that Mama was lost and confused. She brought Mama into her house, gave her a glass of water, and called the number on Mama's identification bracelet.

After Daddy got Mama home and they both were settled, he called me on the phone to share what had happened. We agreed that we were blessed to have the good Lord's protection and to have Mama home again unharmed. Daddy rejoiced. I sensed the relief and excitement in his voice, and I imagined a little spring in his step as we spoke on the phone. Once again, another answered prayer.

Scripture Help: "Or suppose a woman has ten silver coins and loses one. Does she not light a lamp, sweep the house and search carefully until she finds it? Moreover, when she finds it, she calls her friends and neighbors together and says, 'Rejoice with me; I have found my lost coin'" (Luke 15:8–9 NIV).

Prayer: Lord, we are lost when we do not look to you! Lord, thank you for the peace and the wisdom you continue to give Alzheimer's sufferers and caregivers when they feel helpless and lost. Calling on you is all we have when our hope and our strength is gone. Thank you, Lord! We look to you and trust you. Every day we need you, Lord. But, there are days when our fears cause us to need you even more. Thank you for holding our trembling and sweaty hand when we are worried and wavering faith. Thank you for being near us and answering our prayers. We thank you for allowing us to have another miraculous testimony of your goodness in an increasingly hopeless situation. Lord, we are very thankful for your unyielding protection. Lord, we are lost without you; thank you for being our guide when trouble comes. Thank you for being our all when we have no clue what to do next. We are lost when we do not look to you! Thank you, Lord. In Jesus' name, I continue to pray. Amen.

Chapter 12:

Dancing Up a Storm!

I'm a teenager trapped in an old body.
— Betty White

One of the things Mama loved to do was dance, dance, and dance. As her Alzheimer's continued to progress, dancing was the one thing that always brought her comfort. Between the years 2008 and 2011, Mama was still able to socialize and go to family gatherings, Daddy would take Mama to the annual Jackson State University Alumni dance. Since Mama and Daddy were alumni, they enjoyed supporting and attending this event each year. Dancing seems to spark memories from the past for all of us. Dancing helped Mama become more alert, and it seemed to free her from the bondages of Alzheimer's for those moments. Mama was filled with joy and laughter when she danced; dancing had a way of making Mama whole once again. When she was dancing, we all briefly forgot the affliction of Alzheimer's disease. When Mama began to dance, the atmosphere in the room would completely change. In those moments, she regained her self-worth, and the dancing amplified her inner-strength.

As we continued to bring Mama to family gatherings and events, she would usually lead everyone to the dance floor. At larger events, many in the room didn't know Mama was suffering significantly from Alzheimer's disease; she was convincing in spite of all of her other inabilities. For example, my wife, Jeannie, had a graduation celebration at the Thaxton in downtown Saint Louis—an event with approximately 150 in attendance—and Mama led the "Soul Train Line."

As Mama's Alzheimer's progresses, my memories often take me back to places far into my past. I remembered being a kid and Mama playing a stack of 45 records on the stereo; a 45 was a 7-inch fine-grooved vinyl record playing at 45 rpm. This was often a daily ritual for us. In the 1970s, new dance fads appeared almost every week, and we would learn them all. We did the funky chicken, the penguin, and the bump.

I remembered Mama really enjoying one dance in particular. My uncle Howard was always going to the record store to purchase the newest releases. One day, Uncle Howard brought home several 45s he just picked up from the record store in Greenwood, Mississippi. He came in the house grinning, as usual. Uncle Howard said, "Look at what I got." Mama looked in the bag and yelled, "Howard got 'Push and Pull' by Rufus Thomas!" Everyone quickly gathered in the living room. At the house were my sister Iris, Aunt Mary Ann, Cousin Poncho, Uncle Bo, Uncle George, Uncle Lee, Mama Mary, and Papa Johnnie. We all were having our own version of "Soul Train" in my grandparents' living room. Uncle Lee yelled out, "Daisy is dancing up a storm!"

Shortly after he made the comment, the sky got dark and it began to rain hard. Uncle Bo went outside to see what the weather was doing. He frantically ran back in the house and said, "Tornado is coming, and we all are gonna die! Run for your lives!" Of course, no one believed him. We all went outside, and we could see a tornado on the horizon. My grandparents turned the radio on, huddled everyone in the hallway, and closed all the bedroom doors. While we all huddled together on the floor, Uncle Bo whispered in my ear, "I told Papa Johnnie he should have built a storm cellar, and now we're all going to die!" The light in the hallway went out, there was complete silence and we heard a loud roaring sound like a train. After a while, it got very quiet; the wind and the rain stopped in an instance.

After the storm passed, we returned to the living room. To our surprise, the storm had blown out the living room picture window. Then we all went outside to survey the collateral damage. The storm had blown the porch furniture clear off the porch. In addition, the two swings, which had been secured to the ceiling, were blown more than one hundred yards away into the vegetable garden near the smoke house. It was an incredible sight to see, and it all happened in minutes! I guess Uncle Lee was right; Mama did dance up a storm! Uncle Bo said, "We needed the rain. I was worried about my watermelon patch!" I believe Mama's dancing was an expression of her joy and her thankfulness for the memories she continued to cherish. The music enabled Mama to wander to a time and a place when she could recall a memory on demand. The music allowed her to celebrate love, living, and life.

Mama continued to cherish the love we have through dance. When Mama was dancing, she zoomed to a time and place where there was no Alzheimer's disease. Dancing allowed Mama to show the strength and courage to overcome her fears and confusion, to enjoy life in spite of Alzheimer's disease. Seeing Mama dancing showed me that love does stand the test of time. Her joy in movement to music helped me to realize that the next life we will live remains to be seen. "Mama, I am with you, always!"

Scripture Help: "Praise the LORD. Sing to the LORD a new song, his praise in the assembly of the saints. Let Israel rejoice in their Maker; let the people of Zion be glad in their King. Let them praise his name with dancing, make music to him with tambourine, and harp. For the LORD takes delight in his people; he crowns the humble with salvation. Let the saints rejoice in this honor and sing for joy on their beds" (Ps. 149:1-5 NIV).

Prayer: Lord, I thank you for the artful expression of dance and music. It provides a much needed break from the disease for Alzheimer sufferers, caregivers and family. It has been a tremendous blessing to see an Alzheimer sufferer's face light up, and their attitude and mood changing to joy when they are dancing. What a wonderful blessing!

Lord, I thank you for the memories you allow each of us to reach back and reflect upon. Thank you for the precious memories I have shared with love. Thank you, Lord, for allowing me to remember and appreciate what the family once was. Those moments are such beautiful memories, and they have shaped how I live, love, and laugh today. Our memories are wealthy in love, peace, and happiness. I believe those suffering with Alzheimer's often wander in the moments when they seem so far away from the present. Lord, I am grateful! In your precious son's name, Jesus, I pray. Amen.

Chapter 13:

Mirror, Mirror, Mirror

The ravaged face in the mirror hides
the enchanting youth that is the real me.
— Mason Cooley

After Mama had progressed into another stage of Alzheimer's, she became confused and agitated by her own reflection in the mirror. She would often come and get me when she saw her reflection in the bathroom mirror; she would point to her reflection in the mirror and ask, "Who is the person I always see in the bathroom looking at me?" I replied, "It is you. And the other person in the mirror is me." Mama would try to touch the person she referred to, her reflection, and then she would touch me. After becoming frustrated and afraid, Mama would leave the bathroom. She did not understand why she could not touch the woman in the mirror. The reflection appeared to be three-dimensional, and she thought she should be able to touch it. To her surprise, it was impossible. This predicament went on for months, and the issues with the reflection bothered Mama intensely.

There was a full-length mirror secured to wall in the hallway surrounded with pink ceramic roses with green painted leaves. The ceramic roses were something my wife and Mama painted together in craft classes many years ago. Mama would pass this mirror frequently to get back and forth from the family room to her bedroom.

There were times when Mama was afraid to go to the bedroom alone and would ask Daddy or me to walk with her to the bedroom. Mama was afraid of the reflection she saw in the mirror. In her mind, the reflection was a real person. She was very afraid of this person because it was not a person she could touch. Mama's inability to recognize a mirror was similar to a fulfillment of the Alzheimer's disease. Mama could not fight her reflection, and we could not fight Alzheimer's disease. Eventually Mama had enough of being spooked by her own reflection and decided to take matters in her own hands; Mama wanted something done about the strange woman who always ran up on her in the hallway.

One day Daddy and I were on the phone chatting. While he was talking to me, Daddy heard a loud thump as though something had fallen. Earlier, Mama was in their bedroom napping. He thought she might have fallen out of the bed. Daddy abruptly said, "Daisy must be up, and something has fallen. I will call you later!" Daddy hurried toward their bedroom and discovered that Mama had detached the mirror in the hallway from the wall. Subsequently the mirror was broken and she gave the broken pieces to Daddy as she walked down the hall toward the kitchen. Her comment to him was, "I have taken care of the situation; the woman running up on me in the hallway is gone once and for all." Daddy immediately took the broken mirror to the garbage outside. We finally understood how provoking mirrors were to Mama at this stage of the disease.

I find it remarkable that despite Mama's confusion, she always found a way to overcome her fears. There were other mirrors in the house, and Daddy and I were wondering if we would have to remove them all. We both thought it would be weird not to have any mirrors. As her Alzheimer's continued to progress, Mama seemed to no longer be spooked by mirrors; her new approach was to not look in the mirror.

As was normal for Alzheimer's sufferers, Mama had difficulty interpreting visual images and spatial relationships. Mama had reached a point where she no longer recognized her reflection. To Mama, the reflection in the mirror was a real person, not a reflection, and the person in the mirror was a stranger.

Of the two types of memory—short-term and long-term—short-term memory was the first to go for Mama in her Alzheimer's disease. The memories normally stored in short-term memory and later transitioned into long-term memory were no longer possible for Mama. Alzheimer's progressively destroyed this process for her. As Mama aged and her appearance changed, she no longer recognized her reflection. Because she had no short-term memory, Mama did not know what she looked like in the present; so she was afraid of her reflection. Yet, the understanding of a mirror in longterm memory remained. The inability to retain memory prevented the recognition of a mirror; therefore, she saw her reflection as another person she could not reach out and touch. Since she could not understand what was happening, she became afraid, as is normal human nature.

As it is for all Alzheimer's patients, Mama's long-term memory would also diminish—from right to left. The most distant memories were the most accessible to her and the easiest memories to recall. Alzheimer's would fragment her memory until Mama's memory was too impaired for consciousness, and she would decline to a vegetative state.

Mirrors primarily reflect light; the Bible has the likeness of a mirror. The Bible helps us evaluate or measure ourselves. It is a blessed privilege to have the mind, which allows us to remember scriptures to help us understand and identify how we measure up to God's righteousness.

It bothered me that Mama no longer used a mirror anymore; looking into a mirror brought her unbearable confusion. It bothered me that Mama could no longer read a book or watch TV and make sense of it. How could I help Mama in this new progression of the disease? I had to go deeper into the Word of God and learn what God would have me do to exhibit more of what God is.

Scripture Help: "Do not merely listen to the word, and so deceive yourselves. Do what it says. Anyone who listens to the word but does not do what it says is like a man who looks at his face in a mirror and, after looking at himself, goes away and immediately forgets what he looks like. But the man who looks intently into the perfect law that gives freedom, and continues to do this, not forgetting what he has heard, but doing it—he will be blessed in what he does" (Jas. 1:22–25 NIV). James describes God's Word as a mirror. The mirror enables us to see our image and allows us to evaluate or measure our image. The mirror in scripture contains the very breath, the very life of God (2 Tim. 3:16 NIV). The spiritual mirror in the Bible reveals two things. First, it reveals who we are presently, and second, whose image we are being conformed to (Rom. 8:29 NIV). After meditating and spending more time in prayer and studying, I am more accepting of God's final authority in all of our lives. God will continually conform us to the image of Christ. Perhaps my experience with Alzheimer's disease in my family is a sacrifice to conform my image more into the image of Christ. Perhaps there are some extraordinary parallelisms with Mama no longer looking into mirrors and me looking into the Bible scripture and evaluating my image and comparing my image to the image of Christ. I find it fascinating how God can use any situation to breathe life and provide divine instruction for learning; this shows how magnificent he really is.

Prayer: Lord, help caregivers to observe and understand what Alzheimer sufferers see as new interpretations of reality as the disease progresses. The symptoms are ever changing. Yet, you are helping me to understand them better each day. Lord thank you for helping me understand that your Word, the Bible, is like a mirror I need to look into every day because you are the source of all of my help. Lord, thank you for showing me how to be a conqueror and thank you for flooding my heart with your patience and kindness. My patience and kindness has been renewed; they have been revived in a way that can only be the instruction and correction of the Holy Spirit. I now have a level of patience and kindness that was not with me prior to my experience with Alzheimer's disease. Thank you, Lord, for the work you invested in me. In Jesus' name, I pray. Amen.

Chapter 14:

It Is Just My Imagination Running Away with Me

Normal is just a cycle on the washing machine.
—Whoopi Goldberg

nother common characteristic of Alzheimer's patients as the disease progresses is inappropriate or questionable behavior. Often, the behaviors are challenging for caregivers, family members, and others to adapt to and process. And they are considered by most to be inappropriate, outrageous, or shocking. When Alzheimer's sufferers are experiencing the later stages of the disease, it is common for them to express anger, rage, argumentative tendencies, cursing, and stubbornness or willfulness. Alzheimer's patients often reserve their worst behaviors for those with whom they are closest, such as a spouse or family members, and such behaviors are usually absent in the presence of strangers.

In Mama's case, I observed delusional and paranoid behaviors with hallucinations about people, places, and things. We had to sometimes simultaneously deal with psychotic symptoms while attempting to provide care, transport her to appointments, or calm her in the midst of an episode. Most times, there was no rational basis to Mama's psychotic attacks. And frequently, I was not aware of the potential catalyst to the episode. Mama's mental wandering and overreaction created situations in her mind, and the rules she lived by were ever-changing. Sometimes, the behavior was dangerous. Most times, it was distressing to those around her, and frequently, it appeared to create depression, confusion, and anger in Mama.

There was no rhyme or reason to her behavior. What made her angry or frustrated one day would make her laugh the next. What made her laugh or smile moments ago would send her into a verbal and physical rage just a moment later. Mama received prescriptions from doctors for a variety of anti-psychotic pharmaceuticals in an effort to manage her unpredictable behavior. For us, using these new drugs was a definite turning point because the alternative would have been to institutionalize her. The other side of this decision, however, was that the medications had unfortunate and seriously destructive side effects. While the medications minimized the psychotic symptoms and provided generally calm behavior, it also produced marked differences in her mental processing, physical agility, and awareness.

If I heard, "Mama is not having a good day," I already knew what that meant. The phrase became part of our daily lexicon and was often used not only to describe what condition she was in, but what kind of resources Daddy and I would have to draw upon to handle what was to come on this day.

Mama's sudden outbursts of rage continued and often had us all on the edge of our seats, particularly at any of our family gatherings. At times, things would seem to be going normal when Mama would have a bout of paranoia or a psychotic attack, and we would be in for a real surprise. It was hard to tell what would set her off, or what she would want to do about the information she was desperately trying to process. She was trying to manage the influx of data, recollections, facts, and new stimuli, but she was using a brain damaged by the effects of this disease. As such, it was not a trustworthy instrument. On some level, it seemed apparent she understood what was going on, which might have been why she would get so upset.

We did learn that when we noticed Mama's anxiety levels spiking, this was a clear indicator an episode was about to begin. As Mama's Alzheimer's progressed, it actually became easier to determine when episodes were most likely to start. Around 4:00 p.m. seemed to be the time when much of her hallucinations and paranoia would be at its greatest levels. Our behavior adapted to ensure we would have Mama headed back home by 4:00 p.m., and this changed the way we socialized, managed appointments, or handled other necessary business. I learned that this change in behavior—the onset of paranoia, delusional behavior, or hallucinations in the late afternoon or early evening hours—was called sundown syndrome for Alzheimer's patients.

Mama also exhibited hoarding tendencies. In particular, she seemed to hoard books. Mama had an extensive book collection that had amassed over the years. After sunset, Mama would spend hours moving books from one area to another. Sometimes, she would select a book and act as though she was reading it. Even though she had long lost her ability to read and process written language, she appeared determined to try. She also didn't realize how language should look. As a result, many times she would hold books upside down and attempt to make sense of what she was seeing. The one book I noticed she selected more often than others was her Bible. When I saw she was attempting to read her Bible, or when I noticed she was getting frustrated, I would take it from her and read it to her. She would usually sit back and listen, although I was not sure if she was able to comprehend or retain what she was hearing.

I believed Mama knew she was losing her ability to read and write some time ago. I gave Mama an olive wood Bible in a praying hands stand made of olive wood along with an olive wood cross I purchased from Jerusalem in the summer of 1985. In 2007, Mama asked me to take the olive wood Bible with the praying hands and she said she would keep the cross. At the time, I did not understand why she was giving me this, but eventually I did.

Mama's new behaviors also included swearing like a sailor. This was completely out of character for Mama, who always carried herself like a lady and never used this kind of language in her younger days, even when she was angry. Daddy would be in amazement at this change in his wife. He would say, "When did she learn to talk so bad? Where could she have picked up all this cursing?" Sometimes she would say curse words out of anger, and other times, she would say them in a matter-of-fact way and laugh. In a twisted way, some of it was actually timely and funny. She would sometimes have us all in stitches, and she would laugh and ask, "What is so funny?" As her Alzheimer's progressed, her feisty behavior became more and more amplified.

There was another incident when Mama was visiting my house and having a nice conversation with her younger sister, Aunt Mary Ann. Suddenly, Mama accused Aunt Mary Ann of taking something from her, and she wanted it back. Aunt Mary Ann tried to tell Mama she did not know what she was talking about and did not have whatever it was Mama thought she took. Mama raised her voice and said, "You know what I am talking about, and I want it back now!" Then Mama grabbed a large knife my wife, Jeannie, was using to slice ham and began chasing Aunt Mary Ann with it throughout my house. Aunt Mary Ann screamed and ran to get away, and Mama followed close behind her. It was like a horror movie unfolding before our very eyes. I sprang into action and intercepted Mama, taking the knife from her. Mama broke down in tears, and the family stood still, paralyzed from shock. Aunt Mary Ann was shaking, terrified by the episode.

Quickly, I took Mama outside for a long walk through the neighborhood in an attempt to calm her down and to get her to change her focus to something more pleasant. We returned to the house later and Mama was behaving normally, as she was just before the incident occurred. While everyone else was still a bit rattled and Daddy seemed to be embarrassed, I felt it was important to move us all past this episode. "Relax, Daddy, I got this. Relax…enjoy yourself," I told him as I eased Mama into a chair and sat with her. Daddy exhaled and sat back in his chair, maintaining a watchful eye on his wife.

I had come to believe we had to deal with the episodes as they came. If we worried about each episode and let our own fears take control, then Alzheimer's would win again. It could not win! As a family, we had to find humor in all situations so we could hold on to our joy. Our strength was in our joy. I decided that whoever said laughter was the best medicine could very well have been correct. By trying to maintain a lighter mood, all of us could adapt to the changes when they were sure to continue to come our way. We had to avoid resenting Mama for things that were so obviously outside of her control.

Scripture Help: "Though the fig tree does not bud and there are no grapes on the vines, though the olive crop fails and the fields produce no food, though there are no sheep in the pen and no cattle in the stalls, yet I will rejoice in the LORD, I will be joyful in God my Savior. The Sovereign LORD is my strength" (Hab. 3:17–19 NIV). Why is joy important? Because "the joy of the Lord is our strength" (Neh. 8:10 NIV) Joy produces strength. In addition, strength is needed to fight, and Alzheimer's indeed is a fight that tests our faith. We oftentimes struggle to fight because we have lost our joy.

Prayer: Lord, I am tired; it seems like this Alzheimer's is always winning! I need your guidance. Lord, I need more of you! I need more joy so I can remain strong and not wither. I need more of your peace, your kindness, and your gentleness. I face many trials every day, and I do my best, yet it seems like my best is never enough. There are always people who are never happy with my performance. Complaints and criticisms are often crowding my thoughts; at times, it is all I can hear and can be so discouraging. I am overwhelmed with negativity. I feel like nothing I do is ever good enough. Help me not to be discouraged; help me to be always encouraged. Caregivers are tired, and it is written all over their face. Lord, restore the caregiver's joy and their strength. Help us all to honor their sacrifices as they provide care for Alzheimer's sufferers. At times, it just seems like everything I am facing is impossible. Help me, Lord, to see beyond all of the impossibilities and to lean on you. Lord, I do not want to ever stop believing and trusting you. Lord, do not let me become empty. Lord, keep me filled and full of your Holy Spirit. Help me to understand what it is I need to understand. Help me, Lord, to have the strength required to always move forward and continue this battle to the end. Lord, I do not want to throw in the towel; I do not want to ever give up. Lord, cheer me up, comfort me, and make me smile. Lord, I can really use a good laugh. Show me the humor in it all, even when I do not see it for myself. Lord, help me to trust you with everything and doubt you for nothing. Today, I thank you for listening to me! I love you! In Jesus' name, I pray. Amen.

Chapter 15:

Safe House

Safety's just danger, out of place.
—Harry Connick Jr.

Growing up, our house was the Kool-Aid house. Our house was where everyone wanted to hang out and have fun; it was the cool house. Mama had a ton of nieces and nephews. Because Mama was everyone's favorite aunt and sister, she had an extensive collection of photographs, glamour shots, souvenirs, and artifacts from family and friends who had traveled throughout the country and world. Family and friends enjoyed giving Mama keepsakes because she genuinely appreciated and treasured anything people gave her. As a result, keepsakes covered the walls, shelving, and tabletops throughout the house.

Mama was a devoted homemaker; she made the home a safe haven that was comfortable, filled with Southern hospitality, and more. But Mama's behavior had changed because of her psychotic symptoms, such as hallucinations, delusion, and paranoia. The accelerated progression of Alzheimer's disease made Mama and Daddy's house seem more like Amityville horror than the Kool-Aid house. We had to rethink and reconfigure the entire house to make it a home Mama and Daddy could live in and function. Mama's paranoia was becoming more intense, resulting in more mood swings and outbursts of violence.

Mama's paranoia attacks were intense, and Mama was not able to think rationally. At times, she would go into a violent rage or simply a state of such confusion that she could hurt herself or someone else. We had to identify anything and everything that could possibly be a weapon and store it behind lock and key. When she was paranoid, she believed someone was trying to bring her harm. She felt as if someone was trying to take her purse or sexually assault her; her natural instinct was to fight or pick up anything she could use to defend herself.

We locked up cleaning supplies, removed locks from all interior doors, including the bathrooms, and took out dangerous items from medicine cabinet. Mama would think a bottle of Pine Sol was a liter of lemonade or a bottle of window cleaner was Kool-Aid. Daddy installed a shut-off valve on the gas stove so he could cook without worrying that Mama would turn on the stove and burn herself or create a natural gas hazard and blow up the house. For months, Mama would stand in the kitchen as though she were cooking and washing dishes. Eventually, she gave up the cooking attempts because she could never get the stove to come on. Later she would try hard to wash dishes. She was able to make the water come on, but she could not use the dishtowel to clean the dishes.

Another way we tried to limit the chaos was reducing Mama's wardrobe; Mama had many clothes, and they all became much too big for her due to her dramatic weight loss. She often wore several outfits at the same time. I would often see Mama with three pairs of pants, three skirts, and six matching tops. We constantly wrestled with her to get her into just one outfit instead of seven outfits.

We also had to remove nearly all the pictures from the walls as well as Mama's collections of statues and whatnots. The wall hangings seemed to cause many of her hallucinations and paranoia, which manifested into frustration and outbursts of violence. She said the photographs were out to get her and she heard their voices when she passed by. She would often cry, "Someone help me, please!" as she sobbed and shook with fear.

It was also a major problem that Mama was rapidly losing her spatial-awareness. Mama had lost her ability to distinguish what was real what was not real, such as reflections in the mirror or images on the television. She would believe scenes on the television were really happening, and she was included in the scene or program. Scenes that portrayed violence or intense arguing would upset her and she would try to protect herself or shout at the television.

Sadly, all the things that used to bring a smile to Mama's face were now tormenting her. Mama and Daddy's home had become their private torture chamber. Ironically, what became real for Mama became real for all of us. The process of safe-proofing Mama and Daddy's house was an eerie experience for me. It felt like we were packing up Mama's personal belongings as though she had passed away; yet, she was still with us. She didn't understand what was happening and was running around the boxes of clutter like a little kid on moving day.

I was still grieving; packing up Mama's things as though she was gone intensified my grief. I went to the Word of God seeking answers to this ever-changing Alzheimer's journey. God had a purpose for Mama's life that would not end here on Earth. According to Rick Warren (2002), we all spent nine months in our mother's womb to prepare us for life on Earth, and so life on Earth was preparation for life in eternity. As I reflect on Mama's Alzheimer's journey, it changed my values. I was no longer consumed by fear, anger, approval, and possessions anymore. Mama's journey with Alzheimer's gave me a better understanding of how fragile and how short life is. Perhaps I am finally learning God's opinion of me and I am learning my identity?

Scripture Help: "The LORD is my rock, my fortress and my deliverer; my God is my rock, in whom I take refuge. He is my shield and the horn of my salvation, my stronghold" (Ps. 18:2 NIV). "No one will be able to stand up against you all the days of your life. As I was with Moses, so I will be with you; I will never leave you nor forsake you" (Josh. 1:5 NIV). "I give them eternal life, and they shall never perish; no one can snatch them out of my hand. My Father, who has given them to me, is greater than all; no one can snatch them out of my Father's hand. I and the Father are one" (John 10:28–30 NIV).

Prayer: Lord, I am praying for safety and your protection. Lord, please help us to seek you and your righteousness and not the trouble we see. This journey is demanding and grueling. The suffering of Alzheimer's sufferers and caregivers can be overwhelming. Lord, help all caregivers to endure the infirmities of the ones they care for. Lord, unite our suffering with Christ's suffering and use it to witness to others. So they may accept you as their Lord and Savior. Your protection is awesome. We trust you to answer our prayers. In Jesus' precious name, we pray. Amen.

Chapter 16:

The Water

You can't trust water: Even a straight stick turns crooked in it.
— W. C. Fields

*M*ama had developed an incredible fear of water. She would become very afraid when it rained or stormed. Mama would sometimes believe that the garage floor was a huge pool of water. She would often say, "I can't swim; I am not going out there." It would take a lot of convincing to get her out of the house when she genuinely believed the sidewalk or driveway was a pool of water. The fear of water got even worse after 4:00 p.m., making it difficult to wash her hands, wash her hair, or give her a bath.

We found that bathing was one of the most challenging parts of Alzheimer's care giving. Daddy hired in-home healthcare professionals to give Mama a bath, but it was not as effective as we had hoped, so Daddy and I would sometimes work together to give her bath. After it was over, I think we were more soaked than she was, even though she was the one in the water.

Thanksgiving Day, I stayed with Mama so Daddy could travel out of town to Mississippi to spend Thanksgiving with his siblings and their families. It was great for him to get away and spend time with his extended family for an occasion besides a funeral. This holiday was my first time giving her a bath without Daddy's help. I was afraid of the unknown; I prayed my way through it all. I managed to get Mama undressed; it was challenging, but I got through it. Next, I had to get her in the tub and soaped down; to my surprise, it was not so bad. But, Daddy usually washed her private area; I began to pray out loud, "Lord, you know I am not comfortable doing this part. Help me, Lord!" Unbelievably, Mama took the towel from my hand and began to wash herself. I replied, "Thank you, Jesus!" I rinsed Mama off with the shower-head and gave her the towel. She dried herself off. After Mama's bath, I got her partially dressed I applied lotion to her arms, legs, hands and feet. Mama enjoys this part of getting dressed; I give her a mini massage while I am applying the lotion.

Next, I put on the tan outfit Daddy recently bought for Mama to wear on Thanksgiving Day. It was a tan pants suit with a jacket decorated with brown buttons and a large belt buckle that accented her small waist. Underneath the jacket, she wore a brown shell. Daddy always had great taste and he enjoyed buying Mama nice things to wear. The outfit was stylish and comfortable and aligned with Mama's taste. No outfit is complete without the perfect pair of shoes; Daddy and I recently took Mama to Macy's and fitted her for a couple pairs of ankle boots. The pair I put on Mama was brown with a buckle that matched her outfit with a two-inch heel. Finally, I sat Mama on the side of the bed and I combed her hair. She always enjoyed getting her hair combed; I parted her hair down the middle, made two braids on the side, and joined the two braids to the braid I made in back. I put a little makeup on her face and lipstick on her lips and we were done. I combed a lot of hair when my daughter, JJ, was a little girl. I enjoy combing Mama's hair; it is the one activity we can do together.

The next challenge was getting Mama in the truck; sometimes it was a fight to get her in a vehicle, especially when it was cold outside. But this time, she walked outside and got in without any problems. After arriving at my house, Mama got out of the vehicle with no challenges; my wife, Jeannie, got Mama out of her coat, and we all sat on the couch together. Mama was laughing and smiling; she was calm and happy. After sitting for a while, Mama got up and yelled, "Daisy is still here. I am still here!" Mama circled the room with excitement and said she was ready to eat, and that was our Thanksgiving dinner with Mama.

Scripture Help: The Bible enumerates these virtues: "And now these three remain: faith, hope and love. But the greatest of these is love" (1 Cor. 13:13 NIV). "Each one should use whatever gift he has received to serve others, faithfully administering God's grace in its various forms. If anyone speaks, he should do it as one speaking the very words of God. If anyone serves, he should do it with the strength God provides, so that in all things God may be praised through Jesus Christ. To him be the glory and the power for ever and ever. Amen" (1 Pet. 4:10–11 NIV).

Prayer: I pray for all caring for loved ones suffering with Alzheimer's disease. It is so challenging. Give them the needed rest and relaxation they require to continue. Lord, help us to be sensitive to their needs and employing patience and kindness. Alzheimer's robs their victims of so much; therefore, I do not want to be in any way impatient or become frustrated while providing my support. I pray to the Lord for the strength and the courage to honor and respect both the caregiver and the sufferer of Alzheimer's. I thank you, Holy Spirit, for teaching me and helping me to exhibit your love and kindness on this journey. In Jesus' wonderful name, I pray. Amen.

Chapter 17:

Coconut Cake

It is sheer good fortune to miss somebody
long before they leave you.
— Toni Morrison

Mama's four-layer coconut cake was my favorite cake, and she always made me my very own cake for my birthday. Everyone loved Mama's coconut cake; at Mama's annual New Year's dinner, it was the first dessert devoured. Mama would sometimes have to make two so there would be leftovers for family members to take home. As a child, I would sit and watch Mama grate fresh coconut using an old box grater. I loved watching Mama crack the coconut and make the icing. After cracking the coconut, Mama always gave my sister, Iris, and me a little sample of the coconut juice. After Mama finished making the icing, she would give each of us a beater so we could lick the homemade white frosting. These memories of my mother in the kitchen baking her signature coconut cake always bring me great comfort and a smile. Many of my fondest memories of Mama are in the kitchen.

Daddy's eldest sister, Aunt Helen, had recently purchased a new home, and all of the sisters set a date and came to Saint Louis to celebrate. Daddy had five sisters: Helen of St. Louis, Missouri, Nancy and Lynn of Lexington, Kentucky, Marie of Miami, Florida, and Elaine of Anguilla, Mississippi. All of Daddy's sisters coming together to celebrate Aunt Helen's house-warming was a very exciting and historic event for the family; they had never been together in Saint Louis all at once.

The family gathering was not complete without Daddy's double first cousin, Shirley. They were double first cousins because two sisters married two brothers. Cousin Shirley had five brothers and no sisters and Daddy's sisters and Cousin Shirley grew up together like sisters. I always referred to Cousin Shirley as Aunt Shirley because she was the same age as my parents and she just seemed like my Aunt. Aunt Shirley was an exceptionally pretty woman like Mama. She had a light-brown complexion and sandy-brown curly hair. Aunt Shirley was married and they had three children; their names were Aletrice, James Jr. and Sharon. I was close to her children growing up; they were like my siblings. Aunt Shirley's daughter Aletrice and I were the same age, her son James Jr. was two years younger than I was and her youngest Sharon was four years younger than I and was a New Year's baby. When we all were young children, Aunt Shirley and Mama were Girl Scout Leaders together; they would often share in the responsibilities of picking any of us up from various activities. We had a ball growing up together and getting into all kinds of mischief.

After Mama's Alzheimer diagnosis, Aunt Shirley would often call to check on Mama's condition. In our many conversations on the phone, she would often say, "Baby, it simply breaks my heart to see your Mama sick with Alzheimer's. Baby, I am so forgetful at times, I wonder if I have Alzheimer's." I would often reassure her that she did not have Alzheimer's. I enjoyed talking to Aunt Shirley because she was funny and most of all she was a realist. She was probably the only person that would ask me how I was coping with Mama's illness. I really appreciated her asking; I needed someone to show concern for me.

Aunt Shirley was so excited about the family gathering at Aunt Helen's house. She called me several times to get directions to Aunt Helen's new house and that was to be expected. Aunt Shirley was a little ditsy even when I was a kid. However, she was the sweetest and most loving person. I remember when we were kids outside playing and she was on her way to the grocery store. She asked all of us to stand on the porch while she slowly backed her beautiful gold

Fleetwood Cadillac car out of the garage puffing on a cigarette. My cousin Aletrice realized that Sharon's bike was left in the driveway and she made every attempt to get Aunt Shirley to stop the car so we could move the bike out of her way. All of us were on the porch screaming and waving for Aunt Shirley to stop the car. She looked at us on the porch, as though we all were being silly and waved good-bye. She proceeded, and drove the car over the bike. The bike was crushed and the handlebars was caught on the under carriage of the car. We all ran to sidewalk and watched Aunt Shirley drive down the street with a trail of sparks flying from the bike as the vehicle dragged the bike 100 feet. She never once stopped or slowed down as she drove down the street. Eventually the bike separated into several pieces, leaving a trail of parts before finally separating from the underneath the car. It never occurred to Aunt Shirley that we were not waving good-bye. After returning from the store with her groceries, Aunt Shirley asked, "Baby, what happened to Sharon's bike?"

Finally, Aunt Shirley put Alexis, her granddaughter, on the phone and we worked together to get Alexis, Aunt Shirley and her grandson, Nicholas, safely to Aunt Helen's house for the house warming celebration. The house-warming party was going to take place around 4:00 p.m. By this time, Mama had started exhibiting symptoms of sundown syndrome, when the internal biological clock among people with Alzheimer's got out of synch and confusion and agitation would increase around sunset (Smith, G., 2011, April 28). Daddy had become adamant about having Mama back home before 4:00 p.m. because of the sundown syndrome. A few days before the house-warming party, Daddy became hesitant about Mama to the party. I reassured him everything would be okay and Jeannie, my wife, and I would both be with him. I was convinced that between the three of us, Mama would do just fine.

We parked my parents' vehicle in front of Aunt Helen's House. Daddy's twin sister, Aunt Nancy, was in the yard waiting to greet us. After Mama walked into Aunt Helen's house, Mama threw her hands up in the air and said, "I am sorry. I don't remember who anyone is, so don't ask!" Mama shrugged her shoulders and sat down at the kitchen table. I found it to be an incredible response for someone who could not remember my name two hours ago.

Daddy's sisters gathered around Mama, holding her and hugging her, and began introducing themselves to her. Aunt Nancy put her arms around Mama and shared memories of things they had done together. Suddenly Mama remembered. Mama replied, "I know who you are! You are Nancy!" Mama grabbed Aunt Nancy tight; it seemed liked Mama was released from the prison of Alzheimer's for a brief period. Mama remembered each of them and they each had a moment with Mama without Alzheimer's.

We feasted on the incredible barbecue Aunt Helen had prepared, and then Aunt Lynn finished the dinner with her spread of desserts. Aunt Lynn was very skilled at baking; she had baked several cakes. I requested my favorite, a slice of coconut cake. After taking a couple bites of the coconut cake, I realized I had not had coconut cake since Mama had stopped cooking. To my surprise, it tasted exactly like Mama's signature coconut cake. Later I learned from my uncle Glen that Aunt Lynn may have gotten the recipe from Mama Margaret, Daddy's mother. Mama and Mama Margaret often exchanged recipes, and coconut cake must have been one of those recipes. This family gathering could not have been more perfect. After the house-warming party, Aunt Lynn started sending coconut cakes to Daddy and me for our birthdays and other holidays. I have come to realize that Mama's coconut cake was an expression of Mama's love and kindness. It was her way of expressing the love of God's Spirit in her heart. This day reminded me of the love and joy Mama always echoed. It is important to cherish the love Mama shared and cherish the life Mama lived and continues to live.

Scripture Help: "But the fruit of the Spirit is love, joy, peace, patience, kindness, goodness, faithfulness, gentleness, self-control; against such things there is no law" (Gal. 5:22–23 NIV). It does not take a lot to raise someone's spirits. It only takes a kind gesture such as a slice of coconut cake filled with love and kindness. "Be kind to one another, tenderhearted, forgiving one another, as God in Christ forgave you" (Eph. 4:32 NIV).

Prayer: Lord, I am so grateful for the special gifts the Alzheimer's sufferers gave to their family long before their diagnosis and the expressions of love still present in their lives. Lord, I thank you for the ability to recall memories created many years ago to comfort me in the times when I needed it most. Lord, thank you for family and friends—for their thoughtfulness and kindness to share kindness; it is so powerful. Thank you, Lord, for family and friends that expressed love and gratitude to us in this challenging journey in our lives. God, continue to bless them and forever keep them. I thank you, Lord, for your example of sharing love, kindness and goodness. In Jesus' marvelous name I pray, Amen.

Chapter 18:

The Invisible Children

The things we truly love stay with us always,
locked in our hearts as long as life remains.
— Josephine Baker

As the disease progressed, Mama would wander physically and mentally. Her mental wandering included hallucinations, or false perceptions, and delusions, or fixed-false beliefs. Mama often hallucinated that she was still a teacher taking care of her students, particularly female students. Daddy would often ask Mama what she was doing with a bowl, bag of chips, or popcorn. Mama would reply in her teacher's voice, "I am giving my students a snack; I promised them a treat if they were good." Daddy often called these little children "demons." In Mama's efforts to nurture and care for these students, she would often make small messes throughout the house. Toilet paper or paper towels would be scattered across rooms. The students seemed to have more control over Mama's behavior than anyone else did. Mama would ask Daddy or me to get things for these invisible children and would get mad if we did not act accordingly. These invisible children, Mama's hallucinations, were just as real to Daddy and me as they were to Mama.

Mama's hallucinations were only limited to her roles as a teacher or caregiver. Mama did have one traumatic experience when she was a teacher at Sumner High School in St. Louis, Missouri. On Thursday,

March 25, 1993, nineteen-year-old Lawanda Jackson killed her ex-boyfriend, seventeen-year-old Tony Hall, with a shot to the back of his head from a pistol. Jackson reportedly became distraught when Hall began dating another girl. She was now serving a life sentence without parole. Amazingly, this story did not get very much coverage.

Mama believed students and teachers never got the counseling or support they needed to move forward in a healthy way. Mama would talk to me about what happened, and I was simply devastated about the events of the dreadful day and the events leading to the moment. Mama always believed that Lawanda Jackson was pregnant by the murdered victim, Tony Hall. Mama believed a miscarriage and rejection from Tony Hall sent Lawanda Jackson over the edge.

Lawanda Jackson, Tony Hall, and the new girlfriend were all students in Mama's class. The memory Mama often talked about was the sound of a gun going off and the screams. One of Mama's students was present when the shooting happened. This girl ran up three flights of stairs to Mama's classroom. She entered the classroom with blood splattered on her face, hair, and clothes; the blood was most vivid on her blouse. After one of the other students commented on the splattered blood, the female student realized and became hysterical. She began to undress and scream in front of the class because she wanted Tony's splattered blood off her.

Mama thought quickly, found something to drape over her and immediately put the classroom into lock-down mode, and called the office. Mama continued to comfort her and the class until the situation was resolved. The hysterical student splattered with blood seeking help in Mama's classroom was a testimony to the kind of relationship Mama had with her students. Mama always had exceptional rapport with her students. Mama believed and always said, "The children just want to know someone loves and cares about them."

The class of 1993 at Sumner High School was a troubling class for Mama; she talked about the students so much prior to the shooting, I felt like I knew them. Now Mama had Alzheimer's and was having hallucinations about the children she taught and cared for. I listened to Mama's hallucinated conversation with the children. It seemed like she was reliving the events of that day. It was obvious Mama had regrets about the shooting; however, she often replayed the weeks leading up to the incident, trying to identify if there were any clues or hints she may have missed that could have changed the deadly events. Perhaps Mama believed she could have done more to prevent this from happening.

Scripture Help: "Knowing that a man is not justified by the works of the law, but by the faith of Jesus Christ, even we have believed in Jesus Christ, that we might be justified by the faith of Christ, and not by the works of the law: for by the works of the law shall no flesh be justified" (Gal. 2:16 NIV). A stronghold is similar to looking in the mirror and not liking the person you see. It is time to forgive yourself and learn how to love the person God has made in you. A stronghold is an incorrect thinking pattern, and it must be torn down in your mind.

Prayer: Lord, you know our innermost thoughts. Alzheimer's sufferers are not exempt to traumas or overwhelming experiences that continue to haunt them as they wander through their memories. Lord, give them peace with their unpleasant memories or unresolved grief. Help them to find peace in whatever it is that causes them to have hallucinations, paranoia and delusions. Lord, bless caregivers with your strength and your patience to be supportive and understanding when these episodes occur. Lord, help me to accept the gift of goodness, faithfulness, gentleness and self-control that only comes through Jesus Christ. Help me to bring glory and honor to him by seeing myself as a new creation; help me to see my past failures as paid in full by the great sacrifice Christ made on the cross on Calvary. Help me to see myself the same way the heavenly Father sees me! Thank you, Lord, for the knowledge and understanding you have given me about hallucinations and delusions. Lord, I thank you for the love, joy and peace we share. In Jesus' holy name, I pray. Amen.

Chapter 19:

Weary and Burdened

How far you go in life depends on your being tender with the young, compassionate with the aged, sympathetic with the striving, and tolerant of the weak and strong. Because someday in your life you will have been all of these.
— George Washington Carver

*M*ama's Alzheimer's has progressed to a stage I have never seen before. She rarely speaks, and she has lost control of her bodily functions. She now wears adult diapers. The inappropriate, outrageous, or psychotic attacks have not surfaced for quite some time. I believe she has progressed to another stage of Alzheimer's disease, miles beyond the negative behavior. Much to our relief, mirrors, pictures, or images no longer spook Mama. For the most part, she is not responsive to the world around her; she seems to be always in deep thought as though she is meditating.

I also believe her vision has declined significantly, causing some impairment with her mobility. For example, shortly after her second episode of dehydration, she began walking into walls and tables. She walked into the patio door in the family room so hard that it left a knot on her forehead. Then later in the evening, she walked into the wall where the full-length mirror used to hang, bumping her head in the exact same place, making the knot on her forehead even worse. She must recognize that her vision has declined because she has slowed her pace significantly when moving about the house. Mama's second dehydration episode followed the first episode two weeks after my birthday. The doctors said it would happen again and may continue to happen; however, that has not been the case. Mama has not had another dehydration episode in months. The medications for her psychotic episodes were dehydrating her.

Before Alzheimer's, Mama was diagnosed with glaucoma, and for years she used eye drops. Now Daddy gives Mama two different kinds of eye drops daily to treat her glaucoma. Because of Mama's inability to respond to an eye examination, the ophthalmologist cannot treat her glaucoma for any new progressions of the disease. I have learned that a patient's feedback is crucial to a doctor's examination of any kind. It is difficult and sometimes impossible to discern symptoms if the person cannot effectively communicate. In Mama's case, she does not verbally communicate at all. I often wonder if this is a choice or if she simply cannot talk. At times, I believe it is more of a choice. Knowing Mama, I believe, in her own way, she is communicating via non-communication. She is saying, "Why bother?"

Caring for a loved one with Alzheimer's is a tremendous undertaking. The amount of attention required can challenge the caregiver's psyche in many ways. Mama's Alzheimer's disease continues to have a profound emotional impact on our family, relatives, and close friends. Earlier in the progression of her Alzheimer's, Mama's abilities fluctuated from day to day and even from hour to hour. The physical demands of caring for Mama have significantly affected Daddy. Daddy is suffering from grief, depression, and physical fatigue, and yet Daddy is the first to say he is OK and that we all will get through this. Daddy is tired; I see it in his eyes. Seeing his exhaustion makes me feel weary and burdened.

I feel like a platinum-card member of the sandwich generation. Caring for children and aging parents at the same time is a bit mindblowing and overwhelming. I say to people that I do everything from pediatrics to geriatrics. Who would ever have thought? I have learned so much as it pertains to both age groups that I often wonder if I could take a test and add another degree behind my name.

I am constantly juggling between the needs of my parents and my children, and this depletes my time and my energy. There is simply too much to do and not enough time in a day to get it all done. At times, my own emotions are upside down and inside out. I have accepted the irrevocable decline in Mama's health, yet I continue to go through feelings of helplessness and hopelessness, loss of appetite, weight changes, and self-loathing.

As I continue to grieve, I have experienced emotional outbursts both privately and publicly. These outbursts have included tears, anger, defensiveness, or over-sensitivity to feedback on everyday situations. I have learned that the effects of Alzheimer's are much more far-reaching than the person afflicted with the disease; everyone related to Mama is somehow affected. Many family and friends have stopped coming around all together or simply limit their visits.

The one thing that troubles me the most about Alzheimer's is the ongoing family reaction to how Mama is cared for day-to-day. According to Daniel Patrick Moynihan, "Everyone is entitled to his own opinion, but not to his own facts" (1995). I love this quote because it sums up much of the conflict that goes on with Mama's day-to-day care. Those who are not involved in Mama's care do not have the right to impose their thoughts and ideas on those of us who are there every day. Nothing upsets me more than to have others judging a situation when they do not know any of the facts to back up any of their recommendations or solutions. What makes it worse is that they seem unwilling to give up any of their time or resources to be of any help or support. Many of them mean well, and their concern exhibits that they care about Mama. However, they are not there with her. Daddy has been there, day-in and day-out, and this is his wife. It is impossible and wrong to separate her care from his care. Many of the hurtful comments are due to lack the understanding of Alzheimer's disease and the lack of time they have spent with Mama. Daddy is already weary and burdened just because of what has happened to him and to all of us. However, the ridiculous judgments made against him and me make the burden much heavier than it already is. Mama has Alzheimer's, yet we still have to live; we all have a life. I know it is Mama's wishes that we do not stop living.

Scripture Help: "Judge not, and you will not be judged; condemn not, and you will not be condemned; forgive, and you will be forgiven"

(Luke 6:37 NIV). Alzheimer's is a very tough disease to face, and when people who say they know the Lord and condemns you in those low moments when you feel a little weak is more than hurtful; it can be devastating. They disrupt your life with their discouraging comments and go back to their un-shattered life. "Judge not, that you be not judged. For with the judgment you pronounce you will be judged, and with the measure you use it will be measured to you. Why do you see the speck that is in your brother's eye, but do not notice the log that is in your own eye? On the other hand, how can you say to your brother, 'Let me take the speck out of your eye,' when there is the log in your own eye? You hypocrite, first take the log out of your own eye, and then you will see clearly to take the speck out of your brother's eye" (Matt. 7:1–5 NIV).

Prayer: Lord, your Word states that there will be many battles we have to fight and endure. However, you also said we would never be alone. Lord, there are times when I feel unsupported; Alzheimer's disease seems more like war than a single battle. Each new stage of the disease is a fight or struggle I tenaciously resist. I continue to be in awe at the inability to make and store new memories. The inability to learn new information is a phenomenon I was not prepared to deal with. Lord, the progression of the disease has a disturbing impact on my mind, body, and soul. There are days I feel completely helpless and alone. Lord, help me not to feel alone. I know you are with me. Help to feel you when my mind takes me far from you. Lord, there are days where I feel like my heart is ripped from my body while it is still pumping. Lord, help me not to be so heartbroken. I continue to be amazed by how a small change in brain function can produce chaos and confusion for the individual and an entire family. Lord, I need your help. Help me to be compassionate, sympathetic and tolerant at the appropriate times. I pray your love will comfort all of us; I thank you for loving me. I thank you for sending your Son, our Lord Jesus Christ, to the world to save and to set me free. I trust your power and grace will sustain and restore our family. Loving Father, please touch me with your healing hands, for I believe your will for me is to be well in mind, body, soul, and spirit. Thank you for loving me. In Jesus' name, I pray. Amen.

Chapter 20:

Happy Birthday

Don't cry because it's over. Smile because it happened.
—Dr. Seuss

Tomorrow would be my birthday, and I would be another year older. I went into my nightstand drawer and pulled out a few birthday cards Mama gave me through the years. I had a small collection of birthday cards I sometimes read when I got lonely for Mama's voice or Mama's thoughts. I enjoyed seeing her handwriting and signature on the cards. It reminded me of the time when I was learning to write cursive and I thought her penmanship was so amazing; I wanted to write just like her. I would practice my penmanship, and I modeled my handwriting after Mama's handwriting. Mama always signed my birthday cards, "Love Always, Mom."

As I continued to study the birthday cards, I remembered that when I was younger she would sign my birthday cards, "Love Always, Mommy." After I became older she would sign my birthday cards, "Love Always, Mom." I love reading the old cards because they help me to recall so many wonderful memories. Now, the cards were more precious to me than ever before. What I missed the most about birthdays with Mama in full form was sitting at the kitchen table with her, sharing some of her signature coconut cake, while she told me about the day she gave birth to me. She always told me the names she had picked out for me. The names were Gregory Conrad

Fitzgerald Roberts, or Norris Lee Roberts Jr. She allowed Daddy to have the final say, and of course, his choice was to name me after him. Today, I was so thankful that thinking of my mama did not make me so sad. Now when I thought of her with or without Alzheimer's, I smiled or laughed.

Today was a great day! I just learned that my dissertation would be published as a book. I had just ordered my cap and gown for my graduation ceremony. I thought about how proud Mama would have been and the things she might have said to me before she developed Alzheimer's. Mama would have been so tickled to have a son with a Doctorate of Education. I do miss the praises she would often give me.

This day I was heading to a business meeting at the Missouri Art Museum at Forest Park. While driving to the meeting, I gave my dad a call just to check in and see how things were going. Everything seemed fine, and Daddy appeared to be in good spirits. I often called my dad before I went into long meetings, just to let him know I would be out-of-touch for while in case he needed to reach me. The meeting was in a large room in the basement of the Saint Louis Art Museum where I could not get a signal on my cell phone.

When I finally left the long meeting, I saw I had no missed calls, messages, or any text messages; this was a relief. I went to my wife's school, where she was the principal. I visited with her briefly before she had to go to some parent meetings. After I got back in my car, I looked at my cell phone to check for messages and realized I had no more battery charge left on my phone; this changed my plans of going to my parents' house to check in with them. I decided against it because I knew it would not be a brief visit, and I needed to have my phone charged and available since Jeannie was coming home late that night.

After I got home, I plugged my phone into the charger and real-ized I had many missed calls from Daddy, my aunt Mary Ann, and my cousin Marilyn. I thought, *What has happened?* It was unusual to get a stream of calls back-to-back; I knew there was something wrong. I took a deep breath and whispered a prayer for strength and peace for the unforeseen trouble. I asked God to help me before I returned any of the phone calls. First, I called Daddy, and there was no answer. Next, I called my aunt Mary Ann. She answered, "Daisy collapsed on the bathroom floor and hit her head pretty hard. The paramedics said she was very dehydrated. You need to get to the hospital right away." I felt my heart drop to my feet. Again, I asked God to help me get through this.

After getting to the hospital, I saw my cousin, Marilyn, in the emergency waiting room. I asked her to tell me what was going on. She began, "Your Daddy could not get in contact with you on your cell; therefore, Aunt Mary Ann called me to help your Daddy get Aunt Daisy to the hospital because he didn't want to call the ambulance. Your Mama collapsed on the bathroom floor and neither of us could lift her to the bed. Your Daddy is with Aunt Daisy now; the nurses are telling us she is non-responsive." Immediately, my listening process began shutting down. I did not grasp much more of what Marilyn said. All I knew was that I needed to see Mama.

All kinds of thoughts rushed through my mind as I hurried to her room. I saw Daddy sitting in the chair on the left side holding Mama's hand. I could tell he had been crying. I saw the relief in his face when he saw me. Shortly after I arrived, Daddy left to have some alone time to process what had happened. I pulled up a chair to the right side of the bed next to Mama and began talking to her and stroking her head and hand to let her know I was with her. To my surprise, Mama responded to my presence with a smile. I thought, *This is strange.* According to Daddy, Aunt Mary Ann, Cousin Marilyn, and the nurse, she was non-responsive.

I then went to the foot of the bed and began massaging her feet through the covers. Mama began murmuring some words and started to laugh. This contradicted everything said to me before sitting with Mama. Mama was responding to my touch and my voice. I continued to talk to Mama; the nurse was outside the door doing paper work and apparently eavesdropping. The nurse came into the room and said, "You do know she is non-responsive and cannot hear you." In this very moment, Mama's smile disappeared immediately. I thought, *Am I delusional?*

Again, when the nurse came into the room to change Mama's IV and check Mama's vitals, Mama's smile disappeared. The nurse said, "I have been with her all evening, and she has not responded to anyone's attempts to communicate." I replied, "I think you are wrong.

She does not know you, and she is choosing not to respond to you. I think she simply doesn't want to be bothered, for whatever reason." The nurse insisted Mama was non-responsive and I was wasting my time trying to communicate with her.

After the nurse left, I whispered in Mama's right ear, "The nurse is gone!" and Mama smiled again. I said, "Mama, why you are playing possum? Open your eyes!" Mama did not respond to my request. I tried to open her eyes myself, and Mama kept her eyes shut tight. Then I knew I was not delusional and Mama was responsive. Mama was deliberately ignoring everyone. I was not sure why she had chosen to be non-responsive to everyone prior to my arrival. I was just happy the Alzheimer's had not progressed Mama into a vegetative state. My emotions went from despair to joy within seconds.

The next morning Daddy and I arrived at the hospital after Mama had breakfast. We went to Mama's room and were alarmed to see the doctor there waiting to talk with us. The doctor was a large Middle Eastern man and very personable with great bedside manners; Daddy and I both appreciated a doctor talking in layman terms. He greeted us with a smile and said, "Good Morning. You must be Mr. Roberts and this is your son? Have a seat." Daddy shook the doctor's hand and replied, "Nice to meet you!" Daddy asked, "So, what is going on?" After we all took our seats, the doctor leaned closer to us and replied, "Mrs. Roberts is in the last stages of Alzheimer's. Mrs. Roberts only has one kidney functioning, and it is functioning at stage four. Stage five is kidney failure." There was a long pause while he waited for a reaction. We said nothing, so he continued, "Your mother's condition is deteriorating, and her prognosis is very poor."

I replied, "What does this mean?" The doctor replied, "Mrs. Roberts seems to be responding well to the treatment for her dehydration today; however, I suspect this will happen again, and her response to treatment in the future may not be so great. Your family will need to make some decisions about what you will do if her kidney functioning drops below fifteen percent. If Mrs. Roberts' kidney functioning fails, she would not be a candidate for dialysis because of her Alzheimer's and her age. Dialysis is painful, and Mrs. Roberts would have to sit for hours at a time. Based on the stage of her Alzheimer's, she would not sit long and she would likely pull out the dialysis tubes."

There was a long pause and complete silence. The doctor continued to explain, "If Mrs. Roberts' kidney functioning drops below 15 percent that would indicate kidney failure. Without dialysis she would likely die within two or three weeks."

Daddy quickly asked, "What do you suggest?" The doctor replied, "Hospice." In this moment, I went into a trance. All I heard was "Wanh, wanh, wanh, wuh-wahn, wahn." The doctor's voice sounded like Charlie Brown's teacher in the animated version of the *Peanuts* comic strip. All I heard was that Mama was dying because the Alzheimer's drugs had destroyed her kidneys, and today was my birthday.

Daddy went to the cafeteria, and I stayed behind to feed Mama her dinner. I do not know what exactly came over me while I was feeding Mama, but I began to sob uncontrollably, and I could not stop. I did not want Mama to see me cry because I did not want to make her upset.

I thought back to just a few weeks ago: I was by myself with Mama in her bedroom. I had just finished combing her hair while she sat on the bed. I was thinking and became somewhat emotionally overwhelmed with all the problems I had been facing—primarily with being unemployed and our financial struggles. In this moment of despair, Mama threw her arms around me and said, "What's wrong?" This was not the response I was expecting. I held her close, took a deep breath, and said, "I do not know what to do anymore, and I am so tired. Mama, I am so tired. Nothing I do is ever enough; no matter how hard I try." She said, "It will be OK!"

In this moment in the hospital, I needed Mama's mothering and encouragement, and she was there! I was not expecting it. I went to the sink to wash my face to stop crying, but the tears and the sadness continued with such force. I was fighting to hold the tears back, but I just could not stop the tears from falling. In this moment, I was completely overwhelmed with grief and reflecting on the many moments that had led to this one.

As I continued to wash my face in the sink, the tears continued to blur my vision. I felt someone entering the hospital room. As I struggled to see my face in the mirror, the tears continued to come. In the corner of my eye, I saw my Aunt Minnie and my Uncle BF had entered the hospital room. Aunt Minnie threw her arms around me to comfort me. She suggested I take a little time to myself. She said she would finish feeding Mama. I abruptly left Mama's room and headed to the elevators. I went to the cafeteria to spend some time alone and try to regroup.

Scripture Help: "In this you greatly rejoice, though now for a little while you may have had to suffer grief in all kinds of trials. These have come so that your faith—of greater worth than gold, which perishes even though refined by fire—may be proved genuine and may result in praise, glory and honor when Jesus Christ is revealed" (1 Pet. 1:6–7 NIV). The Lord is my daily living. I have come to learn that faith is receiving and faith is recognizing what we have received.

Prayer: Lord, I thank you for your presence! Lord, thank you for the comfort you have provided. Lord, we don't understand so much. Help Alzheimer's sufferers and caregivers not to doubt or waiver. I release my life into your hands. Lord, none of us will escape this journey through death. Teach me how to embrace death with faith. Give families and friends the courage and the strength to hold up their love ones as they continue to step closer to seeing you face-to-face. Lord, take away any fear in the heart of anyone suffering with Alzheimer's. Comfort us, as grief seems to overpower us. You are a good, just, righteous, and loving Father. Do not let any of us grow bitter in the mere shadow of death. Lord, pierce our hearts with the joy only you can provide. Give us the understanding only you can give. Whether in death or in life, your will is accomplished and you are sovereign. Lord, give me rest from the despair I am experiencing. Lord, make me know your presence! Keep me ever aware of your loving hand guiding me through all things. In Jesus name, I pray. Amen.

Chapter 21:

Zoom

I never know how much of what I say is true.
— Bette Midler

The following excerpt is from the author's Mother: Another morning has come. I still hope and wait for the impossible, which is to be well again. These days, neither of us is in a hurry to be at work or anywhere. I like the stillness of these mornings. These days, I feel better in the mornings than any other part of the day. Last night, I slept through the night. I did not get up confused and hung over with fatigue. I continue to dream, and my dreams were vivid. Last night I zoomed from time to time and place to place. It was nice to relive those times when I was well. Last night I saw my mother and father. It was Christmas day, and we were having breakfast. Daddy had just finished saying grace when I zoomed in. I smelled the aroma of Mama Mary's homemade biscuits. We were young. I was pregnant with my baby girl, and my sister Mary Ann was in college. My baby boy, Junior, was a handful. He was talkative and busy. This was the year I got him the *Lost in Space* robot for Christmas. Before I had a chance to sit down and enjoy some of Mama Mary's delicious food, I zoomed again.

I was at my home in the suburbs. It was New Year's Day, and I had just finished freezing the homemade ice cream. I got the recipe from my brother, Howard. My cousin Anna Jean was helping me serve the ice cream to the family. There was family everywhere. I went from room to room, and everyone was having a great time, laughing and talking. The doorbell rang, and it was my sister-in-law, Minnie. She worked at the children's hospital and had to work on New Year's Day. As I took her coat and hung it up in the closet, I zoomed again. It was Junior's graduation celebration from college with his bachelor's degree. We all were sitting down at Calicos having a nice meal, celebrating Junior's and Jeannie's commencement. She would soon be my daughter-in-law. At dinner, I ordered a large chef salad. To my surprise, it came in a serving bowl. It was enough salad to feed our entire party of eight. After dinner, Jeannie's Mother, Carol, and I were taking a picture together. After the camera flashed, I zoomed again.

Then I was at the hospital in the neonatal intensive care unit feeding my granddaughter, JJ. She was so tiny, weighing less than a five-pound sack of sugar. She was so little and so sick. While I held her, I prayed she would be fine. Here comes another nurse with my grandson. He was such a feisty little thing. At the moment he was quiet, and still I was able to hold them both. I always wanted to have twins. It seems God blessed me another way; he gave me twin grandchildren. I cannot wait for the time I can take them to McDonald's and buy them a Happy Meal.

I closed my eyes to enjoy this moment and I zoomed again. Now I was at my daughter's wedding. It was at the church we attended when she was little girl. I am a little sad and glad at the same time. My baby is getting married. I love weddings, and most of all I like planning and coordinating them. Iris was stunning in the dress we picked out together. I took one more glimpse of myself in the mirror before I walked to my seat in the church. Huh! I looked fabulous for a middle-aged woman; my dress was a perfect fit. As soon as I crossed the threshold of the church aisle, I zoomed again. This time I am nowhere in particular. It seemed like I was in a garden alone. It was such a peaceful place, with green pastures and a nice breeze.

Last night I had a pleasant dream of my family. I love my family. What is most wonderful about family is they always accept you with your mistakes and weaknesses and continue to love you, no matter what. I am amazed I am able to remember the dream and enjoy the opportunity to reflect on dreams. In this particular dream, I enjoyed remembering the moments I laughed and smiled with my husband, children, and grandchildren. I laughed at the times I would tell Norris, "I never needed him!" There were times he made me so mad we both said mean things to each other. Yet, deep in my heart, I never really meant it. As I ponder on the marriage vows we took—for better or for worse—I get overwhelmed. We both have made mistakes along the way; does any of it matter now? Now I struggle just to remember what I had for breakfast. Now it is difficult for me to put words together. How do we move forward when I cannot remember his name or remember his face? This is not how I wanted my story, our story, to end. Family, there is a part of me that will never forget and you all play a significant role: the memories of me I deposited in you. Treasure our memories and think of them as keepsakes.

Scripture Help: "He will wipe every tear from their eyes. There will be no more death or mourning or crying or pain, for the old order of things has passed away." (Revelation 21:4 NIV).

Prayer: Heavenly Father, hear my prayer, for my suffering is tremendous. These days I am often lost and confused. Lord, I ask you to give me peace in my heart to endure this trial. Lord, thank you for giving me the dignity I desperately want and desire in this time of life. Lord, I ask you each day to shower my family and me with your blessings, your love, and your wisdom. Thank you, Lord, for how you have blessed my family and me. Thank you for your instruction and guidance when we have no clue what to do next. I am often lost in my losses. Yet in you, there are no losses. There are only gains. Lord, please blanket me with your mercy, faithfulness, and gentleness. What a wonderful tapestry for my soul. I look to you for the joy and strength I need to persevere. Lord, take care of my family. They need you more than ever! Thank you, Lord. In Jesus' name, I pray. Amen.

In Closing

*Memories of our lives, of our works and
our deeds will continue in others.*
— Rosa Parks

Feelings of anger, fear, anxiety, guilt, hopelessness, sadness, and vulnerability are common for individuals with a terminal illness diagnosis (Kübler-Ross, 2005). As Mama's Alzheimer disease progressed, my feelings of loss also progressed. I understood and accepted Alzheimer's was a terminal and incurable illness. Nevertheless, I was angry, and as her Alzheimer's progressed, my anger and frustration escalated. I was angry about how the disease robbed a person of dignity and basic life skills. Mama was our family's memory maker. My sadness began after Mama's memory loss became more severe and the ability to have a true conversation with Mama went from infrequent to not at all. I cried a lot and felt the profound loss of all I knew my mother to be.

Sometimes after visiting with Mama and Daddy, I would cry for hours afterwards. It grieved my spirit to see what was happening to my mother, and the grief was unbearable at times. The feelings of fear and anxiety really kept me on edge. I worried about all the things I could not control. I felt like Mama and Daddy's lives were spiraling. It led me to feelings of hopelessness, and I questioned the strength of my faith. The feelings of hopelessness caused me to feel like the pain would never ease. The feelings of vulnerability overshadowed all of the other emotions I was experiencing, and I found myself losing focus with everyday tasks. I often wondered what would become of me. And I often wondered, would this be my fate as I aged? Then I realized I could not allow the spirit of fear to consume my life. "For the Spirit God gave us does not make us timid, but gives us power, love and self-discipline" (2 Tim. 1:7 NIV). Love is what I have chosen to focus on as I move forward. This is when I stopped crying, and I began to use my energy and strength to provide support for Mama and Daddy.

Alzheimer's has robbed Mama of many things that she cherished and loved. Yet, the one thing I am determined not to let Mama be without is my love for her. "Yet I hold this against you: You have forsaken your first love" (Rev. 2:4 NIV). Mothers are their children's first love. Mama is my first love. I will express my love for Mama by physically caring for her needs and simply spending time with her, for as long as I am able to do so. Mama may not ever call my name again, and she may never have the ability to identify my presence. Yet I will continue to hold her hand, wash her feet, kiss her forehead, comb her hair, and clean up after her. I will continue to give her all the love I can give until our time together on this side of glory is no more. I thank you, Lord, for your wonderful gift, my teacher, my provider, my mama. "For I am persuaded, that neither death, nor life, nor angels, nor principalities, nor powers, nor things present, nor things to come, nor height, nor depth, nor any other creature, shall be able to separate us from the love of God, which is in Christ Jesus our Lord" (Rom. 8:38–39 NIV). This book is a blessed gift from God. Mama, I will always love you for who you are, and I appreciate how you have cared for me.

Alzheimer's disease is a thief and a murderer that robs and destroys its victims of their senses, ability to learn, and precious memories. More must be done to stop these senseless murders.
— Dr. Norris Lee Roberts Jr.

References

"Elaine Axelrod," November 30, 2012
http://therapists.psychologytoday.com/rms/name/
Elaine_R_Axelrod_PhD_Philadelphia_Pennsylvania_54853

"Daniel Patrick Moynihan," (2012). December 31, 2012,
Goodreads.com

"E. Kübler-Ross," (2005), *On Grief and Grieving: Finding the
Meaning of Grief Through the Five Stages of Loss*, Simon &
Schuster Ltd

"Rowe et al," *Persons with dementia missing in the community: Is it wandering or something unique?* BMC Geriatrics
2011 11:28.

"Joanne Silberner," (May 12, 2012). *Alzheimer's Patients Turn To
Stories Instead Of Memories*, Shots Health News from npr.org

"G. Smith, (2011, April 28). Alzheimer. December 31, 2012
http://www.mayoclinic.com/health/sundowning/HQ01463

"Rick Warren," (2002), *The Purpose Driven Life*. Michigan:
Zondervan.

"Bette Midler", December 31, 2012, http://www.brainyquote.com/
quotes/authors/b/bette_midler.html

"Betty White," December 31, 2012,
http://www.goodreads.com/
quotes/474598-i-m-a-teenager-trapped-in-an-old-body

"Bill Cosby," December 31, 2012,
http://www.brainyquote.com/quotes/authors/b/bill_
cosby_2.html

"Bill Cosby," December 31, 2012,
http://www.brainyquote.com/quotes/quotes/b/bill-
cosby446434.html

"Cesare Pavese," December 31, 2012,
http://thinkexist.com/quotation/we_do_not_remember_
days-we_remember_moments-the/154115.html retrieved
December 31, 2012

"Dr. Seuss," http://www.goodreads.com/quotes/1173-don-t-cry-
because-it-s-over-smile-because-it-happened retrieved
December 31, 2012

"George Washington Carver," December 31, 2012
http://www.brainyquote.com/quotes/keywords/compassionate.
html retrieved

"Gilbert K. Chesterton," December 31, 2012
http://www.brainyquote.com/quotes/quotes/g/gilbertkc106572.
html retrieved

"Harry Connick Jr," December 31, 2012,
http://thinkexist.com/quotes/harry_connick,_jr.

"Irwin Edman," December 31, 2012,
http://www.brainyquote.com/quotes/quotes/i/
irwinedman127619.html

"Jerry Lewis," December 31, 2012,
http://www.brainyquote.com/quotes/quotes/j/jerrylewis
451544.html

"Joseph Campbell," December 31, 2012,
http://www.brainyquote.com/quotes/quotes/j/josephcamp
384345.html

"Josephine Baker," December 31, 2012,
http://www.goodreads.com/quotes/104197-the-things-we-truly-
love-stay-with-us-always-locked

"Maya Angelou", December 31, 2012,
http://www.goodreads.com/quotes/5934-i-ve-learned-that-peo-
ple-will-forget-what-you-said-people

"Lena Horne," http://thinkexist.com/quotation/don-t-be-afraid-to-
feel-as-angry-or-as-loving-as/360888.html

"Mason Cooley," December 31, 2012,
http://www.brainyquote.com/quotes/quotes/m/masoncoole
396107.html

"Rosa Parks," December 31, 2012,
http://www.brainyquote.com/quotes/quotes/r/rosa-
parks133228.html

"Sophia Loren," http://www.goodreads.com/quotes/128814-if-you-
haven-t-criedyour-eyes-can-t-be-beautiful

"Sylvia Robinson," December 31, 2012,
http://thinkexist.com/quotation/and-like-any-artist-with-no-art-

form-she-became/360443.html

"Toni Morrison," December 31, 2012,
    http://www.goodreads.com/quotes/392832-it-is-sheer-good-for-tune-to-miss-somebody-long-before

"Toni Morrison," December 31, 2012,
    http://www.goodreads.com/quotes/13872-like-any-artist-with-out-an-art-form-she-became-dangerous

"W. C. Fields," December 31, 2012,
    http://www.brainyquote.com/quotes/quotes/w/wcfields151505.html

"Walter Mosley," December 31, 2012,
    http://www.brainyquote.com/quotes/quotes/w/waltermos1440266.html

"Whoopi Goldberg," December 31, 2012,
    http://www.goodreads.com/quotes/114444-normal-is-just-a-cycle-on-the-washing-machine

Bible Versus

1 Cor. 12:25-27 NIV
1 Cor. 13:8 NIV
1 Cor. 13: 4–7 NIV
1 Cor. 13:13 NIV
2 Cor. 4:16–18 NIV
Eccles. 4:9–12 NIV
Eph. 4:32 NIV
Gal. 5:22–23 NIV
Gal. 2:16 NIV
Hab. 3:17–19 NIV
Heb. 4:12 NIV
Isa. 41:10 NIV
Jas. 1:22–25 NIV
Jer. 29:11 NIV
John 21:18–19 NIV
John 21:18–19 NIV
John 16:24 NIV
John 10:28–30 NIV
Josh. 1:9 NIV
Josh. 1:5 NIV
Luke 15:8–9 NIV

Luke 6:37 NIV
Matt. 27:46 NIV
Matt. 14:1–14 NIV
Matt. 7:1–5 NIV
Neh. 8:10 NIV
1 Pet. 4:10–11 NIV
1 Pet. 1:6–7 NIV
Phil. 2:5 KJV
Ps. 55.1 NIV
Ps. 34:17–18 NIV
Ps. 34:17–18 NIV
Ps. 121:1-8 NIV
Ps. 149:1-5 NIV
Ps. 18:2 NIV
Rom. 8:29 NIV
Rom. 8:38–39 NIV
1 Thess. 5:23 NIV
2 Tim. 3:16 NIV
2 Tim. 1:7 NIV
2 Tim. 1:7 NIV
Rev. 2:4 NIV
Rev. 21:4 NIV

CPSIA information can be obtained at www.ICGtesting.com
Printed in the USA
LVOW07s2240131115

462521LV00001B/52/P